EFT Tapping Revolution

Cure anxiety, stress, addictions, pain, and attract love and wealth with the ultimate tapping solution

By best-selling author and renowned EFT tapping practitioner and trainer:

Randal Lawrence

My free gift to you:

Thank you and congratulations on your purchase! To say thank you, I would like to give you a free instructional video that demonstrates how to tap. You can use this video as an aid while you progress through this book. To claim your free gift now please visit my website at the URL below. I hope you find the video helpful:

www.randallawrence.com

More books from Randal Lawrence

Available on Amazon

EFT Tapping and the Law of Attraction
How to eliminate negativity and attract wealth, happiness, love, positivity, and abundance into your life starting TODAY!

EFT Tapping for Weight Loss
Overcome junk food cravings, increase your willpower, speed up your metabolism, and transform your mind and body!

EFT Tapping Miracles for the Soul:
Six inspiring and uplifting stories of positive change and transformation through Emotional Freedom Therapy tapping

Learn EFT Tapping NOW! Complete Beginner's Manual:
Relieve stress and anxiety, lose weight, control cravings and addictions, boost your confidence and self-esteem and attract abundance starting today

Praise for *The EFT Tapping Revolution*

I believe Randal Lawrence is at the forefront of a new healing method that will radically redefine the concept of wellness and the next generation of health care professionals. His simple and methodical approach has helped me to reshape my life around healthy habits and to break the pattern of negative thoughts and self-destructive actions that I used to struggle with. This book will change your life – I know it changed mine!

- Ernesto Delviro, Ph.D., professor of biology

The EFT Tapping Revolution lays out a new vision for what life can be. It is practical in nature, but includes the theoretical background you need to truly understand what tapping is, how it works, and how you can use it to improve your life.

- Jamal Harris, M.Sc., Ph.D., psychologist

What a breath of fresh air *The EFT Tapping Revolution* is! In a world teeming with misery, selfishness, and pessimism, Randal Lawrence delivers a relentlessly positive take on life and getting everything you want out of it. Lawrence comes across as an experienced and knowledgeable friend who is there to guide you through your minor struggles or your darkest hour.

- Ann Mayfair, school teacher

I warn anyone considering reading this book that you may not be able to put it down. I read from cover to cover, excited by the power of tapping and inspired by the touching stories of its real life application that are intertwined throughout this beautiful book.

- Sophia LaFleur, artist and mother

I discovered tapping recently and it changed my life. Since then I've read just about every book there is to read on the subject and I can honestly say that *The EFT Tapping Revolution* by Randal Lawrence is one of the very best out there. Whether you are an experienced practitioner of energy psychology or someone who has never tapped before, I urge you to read this book without delay.

- Abdul Badee Rahman, Ph.D, university professor

Tapping is deceptively simple, surprisingly fun, and disarmingly powerful. Within the first few pages of *The EFT Tapping Revolution* you have learned enough to begin tapping yourself. By the end of the book, you have the knowledge and the training to unlock the raw power of emotional freedom therapy.

- Gary Reese, magazine editor

If you are desperately looking to change your life, do not waste another second looking for an answer to your problems. All you need to know is contained within the pages of Randal Lawrence's latest book, *The EFT Tapping Revolution*.

- Abella Hymans, nutritionist and yoga instructor

It is a phenomenal day when you discover something as simple and powerful as tapping works for you. This is the book that helped me to finally lose the excessive weight I carried for years. Randal Lawrence, I thank you for giving me the strength to be healthy.

- Nick Sinclair, accountant

It is as if Randal Lawrence took everything that is known about psychology, biology, medical science, and human happiness, and boiled them down to a single, practical guide. *The EFT Tapping Revolution* is a blueprint to the good life.

- Lupita Sanchez, author and public intellectual

I admit I was cynical at first that something as simple as tapping could really work, but after applying the techniques taught in this book I am a believer. Tapping has worked for me and it can work for you too. I am a believer.

- Hans Fuhrmann, B.Eng., chemical engineer

I have personally used tapping to cure myself of the debilitating anxiety that I have suffered from since childhood. Nothing else worked and I thought I would live with this condition forever – until I read *The EFT Tapping Revolution!*

- Jessica Craig, web designer

Legal notice

This book is copyright (c) 2015 Randal P. Lawrence. All rights reserved. This book may not be copied or duplicated in whole or in part via any means including electronic forms of duplication such as audio or video recording or transcription. The contents of this book may not be stored in any retrieval system, transmitted, or otherwise copied for any use whether public or private, other than brief quotations contained in articles or reviews which fall under the "fair use" exception, without express prior permission of the publisher.

This book provides information only. The author does not offer any advice, medical or otherwise, or suggest a particular course of action in any specific situation, nor is this book meant as a substitute for any professional advice, medical or otherwise. The reader accepts all responsibility for how he or she chooses to use the information contained in this book and under no circumstances will the author or publisher be held liable for any damages caused directly or indirectly by any information contained in this book.

Table of Contents

More books from Randal Lawrence........................3
About this book..10
Introduction...12
PART I: Tapping basics: start tapping today!............14
What is EFT tapping?....................................15
The 17 key tapping points...............................16
Before you begin tapping................................20
How to tap..24
PART II: Advanced tapping: theory and practice..........29
How EFT tapping affects the brain.......................30
Targeting your tapping..................................36
Developing your own tapping scripts.....................38
Mindfulness...42
The coming paradigm shift...............................44
Affirmations..50
Chakra clearing...56
Blaming others to escape personal responsibility........74
Why isn't EFT tapping working for me?...................78
Tapping for children and teens..........................87
True tapping miracles: The young gangster...............90
PART III: Transform your life with EFT tapping..........95

Mindset shifting for increased self-esteem..........96

Losing weight with EFT tapping..........99

True tapping miracles: the yo-yo dieter..........108

Controlling cravings and addictions..........112

EFT Tapping to Cure Anxiety..........125

True tapping miracles: years of anxiety, cured in minutes 134

Law of Attraction: how to make more money and attract wealth into your life..........138

Law of Attraction: fall in love, improve your relationships, and attract the people you want into your life..........146

True tapping miracles: The young family man headed for divorce..........156

EFT Tapping for rejection and heartbreak..........160

True tapping miracles: The devastating breakup..........166

EFT tapping for pain relief..........170

The most important thing to remember..........177

One final note..........179

More books from Randal Lawrence..........181

About this book

The chapters in this book have been organized in three parts. Part I of this book is the most important for those new to EFT tapping as it teaches the reader how to begin tapping and essentially lays the foundation for everything else that follows in this book. For those already familiar with what tapping is and how it is done, Part I will provide a quick refresher on the current best practices when it comes to the basics of tapping.

Part II of this book leaves the basics of EFT tapping and delves in the more advanced aspects of this therapeutic technique. I will explain some key findings and research data on how EFT tapping affects the brain which will help you to understand how tapping works and what it is capable of. Perhaps the most important chapters in Part II of this book are the two chapters on *Targeting your tapping* and *Developing your own tapping scripts*. These skills essentially teach you how you can most fully benefit from the power of tapping by customizing your approach to achieve the results you desire. I encourage you to refer to these chapters whenever necessary as you proceed through the book as in many ways they contain the keys to move on from the beginner stage and become an advanced practitioner of EFT tapping.

Also in Part II, I will explain the concepts of mindfulness and affirmations and how they relate to tapping. I will also reveal what I believe is a dramatic paradigm shift in wellness and health that is right around the corner. The chapter on the chakras contained in this section of the book will help you deepen your understanding of energy psychology and the included exercise will be of assistance in applying this teaching immediately as you read through the book.

The chapter *Why isn't EFT tapping working for me?* is another must read chapter in Part II of this book that will be of assistance to those who are not immediately experiencing the results they desire with tapping. In my experience, tapping works for virtually everyone but *only when it is applied correctly*! In this chapter I'll explain the three common mistakes that can sabotage the success you want, and show you how to avoid them.

In Part III of this book we will draw on everything you've learned about tapping in Parts I and II to tap through specific problems and challenges. There are specific chapters on many of the most common difficulties people experience in life, such as low self-esteem, weight loss, addictions, cravings, pain relief, anxiety, love, and money.

By the end of this book not only will you be an expert on how tapping works, but you will understand exactly how tapping can be applied to radically transform your own life, as well as the lives of your loved ones.

Introduction

I never thought that I would find myself on the forefront of a movement like EFT tapping. Back when I was a young undergraduate science student, I envisioned my life unfolding in quite a different way. I expected that after many years of study I would go on to work as a scientist, conducting research in a laboratory and perhaps teaching some courses at a college or university. If I was lucky, I might play a small role in researching some new drug capable of saving lives by curing a previously incurable illness.

The thing is, back when I was so deeply immersed in the pursuit of promoting health through science, if you had told me about EFT tapping I probably would have just laughed about it. I had the attitude that a real scientist, doctor, or other medical professional shouldn't be wasting their time with "new age" and "woo woo" stuff like tapping. I thought that modern Western medicine was the pinnacle of health and wellness, and that anything outside of the prevailing allopathic practice was surely just bunk. Boy was I wrong.

It wasn't until I was in my own darkest hour that I was willing to give tapping a try. My long-time girlfriend had just broken up with me, a crucial deadline for some research on my academic thesis was fast approaching, and a close friend had just died suddenly and unexpectedly. Emotionally, I was a wreck. I couldn't focus on anything. It felt like the weight of everything going on in my life was crushing me, as if I was suffocating beneath a mass of sadness, anger, anxiety, confusion, and fear that I was powerless to overcome no matter how hard I tried. It was in that moment that I was finally ready to try something new, even if I didn't understand it. Even if I thought it looked stupid.

I remember that night like it was yesterday. I remember it not because of the turmoil I was experiencing, but because of the sudden and dramatic relief that tapping brought to me. In my first session, in a matter of minutes, I felt the fog in my mind fade away. I felt the intensity of these powerful emotions wither and wane. I had a clear head again. I could focus and direct my mind toward whatever I wanted, no longer a slave to the challenges of the day. I felt like in an instant I had grown 10 miles high and I was just staring down at these tiny little troubles that only moments before had so consumed me.

It was a revelation to me at the time, and yet the real revelation would come in the days that followed. If tapping had so quickly, easily, and effectively worked for me, who else could it work for? And *what* else could it work for? I was so intrigued that from then on I forgot all about working to make the drug companies richer, or contributing to our narrow Western school of thought on health and wellness. I had found a real therapeutic technique that offered dramatic relief to a wide array of common ailments. A therapeutic technique that is completely accessible to anyone willing to take a few minutes to learn how to do it. A therapeutic technique that does not require drugs, money, or any highly specialized knowledge. I had found my calling in life: to share the power of EFT tapping with the world, and also to share this power with you, right now.

I congratulate you on investing in your own health and wellness by reading this book and I am looking forward to sharing with you a new healing movement that I believe will change the world. When you are ready, just turn the page and we'll begin your journey together.

PART I: Tapping basics: start tapping today!

What is EFT tapping?

EFT stands for Emotional Freedom Technique. At its heart, EFT tapping holds that an imbalance or disturbance in the body's natural energy system is what accounts for basically all of the troubles we may suffer from in life. Emotional trauma, destructive habits, and physical pain are all manifestations of an energy system that has become blocked and thrown out of its natural equilibrium.

I find it amusing that people sometimes criticize energy psychology generally, and emotional freedom therapy specifically, as being something that is new, unproven, or radical. The fact that the human body has an energy system and that this energy system is crucial in maintaining whole body health and wellness is neither new nor radical. The ancient Greeks and Romans knew that a balanced energy system was an important part of maintaining one's health. For centuries, many Eastern cultures have also based their healing techniques on facilitating a natural energy flow through the body. One of these healing techniques that has been somewhat popularized throughout the Western world as well is acupuncture. Acupuncture is based on a similar concept as EFT tapping in that it is meant to facilitate an equilibrium in the body's energy system. EFT tapping actually uses the same energy meridians that acupuncture does, however it improves on this older technique in a variety of ways.

Put in a nutshell, EFT tapping works by resolving disturbances and blockages that are inhibiting the natural balance and blow in your energy pathways. By resolving and eliminating the disturbances, EFT tapping restores a calm equilibrium to your body and allows your energy pathways to flow uninhibited the way they are meant to.

The 17 key tapping points

The following points are linked to key energy meridians within your body. These are the spots you will tap on as you go through the various tapping sequences explained in this book.

1. Side of the hand: the part of your hand that would make contact with an object if you were doing a "karate chop". There are two of these points, one on each side.

2. Inside wrist: the middle of your wrist on the same side as the palm of your hand. There are two of these points, one on each side.

3. Top of the head: the point at the very top and center of your head.

4. Eyebrows: the point where your eyebrow begins on the side closest to your nose. There are two of these points, one on each side.

5. Side of the eye: the point right beside your eye, on the bone, and on the side of each eye closest to the ear. There are two of these points, one on each side.

6. Under the eye: the point under the eye just below where the bone begins. There are two of these points, one on each side.

7. Under the nose: the point underneath your nose and above your top lip.

8. Chin: on your chin about one finger length below your bottom lip.

9. Collarbone: the point on your collarbone below your neck. There are two of these points, one on each side.

10. Under arm: The point underneath your armpit near the top of your rib cage. For men this will be even with the nipple. For ladies, this will be even with the bra strap. There are two of these points, one on each side.

For your convenience, a photograph illustrating the 17 key tapping points is included. A dot has been placed over each point. I have also prepared a brief video demonstrating how to tap on each of the tapping points that I would be happy to give you. Please visit my website at **www.randallawrence.com** to access the video for free.

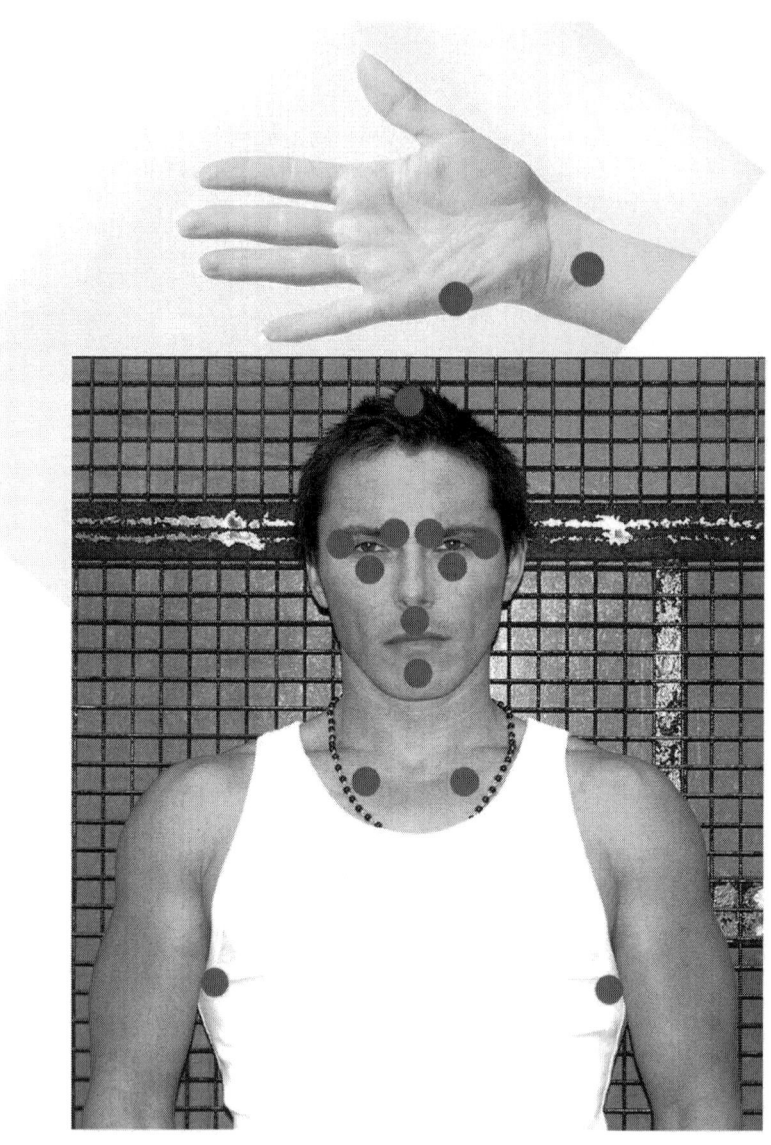

Visit my website at **www.randallawrence.com** to access the free demonstration video

Before you begin tapping

There are a few important steps you can take before you begin a tapping session in order to maximize its effectiveness. Much of this chapter should be taken as suggestions only however. One of the truly great things about EFT tapping is how easy and accessible this technique is to incorporate into your daily life no matter how busy you are. If you are so busy that the only time you have to devote to tapping is while you are stopped at a red light, or while you are on a bathroom break at work, you can still experience amazing results from tapping in whatever place and time you are able to. This chapter is not meant to discourage you from tapping through a problem quickly while you are on the elevator just because you don't have time to sit down, and get comfortable and really in tune with your body. Your results will surely be better if you do follow the advice I'll give you here about preparing to tap, but don't think of these suggestions as absolutely necessary. They are more like icing on the cake, rather than the cake itself.

If there is a persistent problem or issue in your life that you wish to tap on, it is helpful if you can get into a habit of tapping daily. I know many of the people I have met and coached who have had the most success with tapping have set up a non-negotiable daily period of tapping that they adhere to faithfully. Many have a set time, such as after work but before dinner, or first thing in the morning. The first thing to do if you want to commit to achieving success with tapping is to do it regularly. You don't need to devote significant time to daily tapping as each session can be tapped out in only a few minutes. Even the most busy people should be able to spare a few minutes to improve their health and well-being. If you feel you don't have the time for this, I'd encourage you to carefully evaluate the priorities in your life and also to consider how much better off you would be if you could break through the blockages you suffer from by committing to tapping regularly.

Once you've committed to tapping regularly, think about the time of day you will tap. Having a plan for tapping helps ensure that you follow through on your commitment to make this positive change in your life. Of course you can tap in addition to the time you select as well, on days where you feel you can benefit from additional tapping. Initially you'll want to set aside about 15 or 20 minutes for each tapping session. This is a good amount of time for a beginner to get in the habit of tapping and experience its amazing results, without it becoming a burden that takes up too much time.

When it is time to begin tapping, stare by sitting down in a comfortable position. You can sit on the floor, a chair, or even your couch. All that is important is that your spine is straight. You don't want to slouch or lay down. The angle of your spine is very important and in order to maximize the free-flowing energy you are attempting to facilitate, you need to sit up straight. You don't need to be over-focused on your breathing. You can take slow and deep breathes naturally as you move through the tapping session.

Take a moment to clear your mind of any particular thoughts before you begin tapping. Think of this has hitting a "reset" button in your mind, that will clear the slate and prepare you to focus on tapping through your blockages. What will happen is that for a few seconds, maybe 5 or 10, your mind will be clear. But then the thoughts that were previously in your head will slowly creep back in. Before this happens, you want to focus your thoughts on what your body is telling you. Let all other thoughts go. Think about you feel physically. Are you comfortable? Think about where the weight of your body is contacting the chair or the floor and how that feels. Think about your temperature, and take time to notice any subtle sounds or smells around you in your environment.

Slowly turn your attention to your mind and your mental well-being. How are you feeling? How do your arms feel? Your legs? Pay attention to the joints. How do the muscles feel? Do you feel any aches or pains? What about your head, neck, shoulders, and throat? What emotions are you experiencing? Are they connected to what you want to tap on? Begin to direct your attention towards what you will be tapping on. Think about what the issue is. Listen and receive the feedback your body and mind is giving you. Let other thoughts go and focus just on the issue you will tap on. Think about how it is making you feel right now.

When you are feeling focused and self-aware, you need to rate what you are experiencing on a scale of 1 to 10. Suppose that you are going to tap on anxiety. Ask yourself how anxious you are at that time, where 1 is the minimum level of anxiety, and 10 is the maximum, most overwhelming amount of anxiety. Pick the number that best corresponds to your current feeling. Take responsibility for your own emotional well being. Recognize that no other person or situation in the world can control your emotions, feelings, and energy flows better than *you*. It is *your energy*. Take agency and responsibility for it. When you have finished each of these preliminary steps, it is time to begin your tapping session.

How to tap

There a number of different ways to go through an EFT tapping session. The type of tapping script you use will depend on the type of problem you are trying to solve. In this book I will take you through a number of different tapping scripts for common problems. I encourage you, when you are comfortable with the basics of tapping, to develop your own tapping scripts customized to you. This book contains all the information you need to do that. Pay close attention to the chapters in this book about how tapping works, and how to develop your own tapping scripts. Below is a general tapping script meant to calm your emotions and ease any overwhelming feelings. It is a good way to start, but as you learn more about EFT tapping you will want to target your tapping towards specific blockages, as you will learn to do in this book.

If you are new to tapping, you may find it helpful to follow the free video demonstration I have prepared for readers of this book. If you think this would be helpful for you, please visit my website to get access to this free video and use it to help you tap through your first few sessions: **www.randallawrence.com**

Now let's start the tapping sequence. Start by tapping with four fingers on point 1, the side of the hand (or the "karate chop point"). Tap gently. There is no need to be aggressive with yourself or hurt yourself. Say out loud:

"even though I am feeling so much stress, and overwhelming emotions right now, I profoundly and completely love and accept myself. I profoundly love and accept the way I feel right now. I profoundly love and accept myself and everything that I am."

Move on to tapping on point 2, the inner wrist. You can tap with two fingers, four fingers, or your opposite wrist. Say out loud:

"Even though I feel so much stress and turmoil in my life right now. Even though sometimes the stress feels overwhelming. Even though sometimes I feel like I can't focus on anything or function the way I want to because of these intense feelings. Even though I feel this way, I profoundly love and accept myself, and my body, and the way it feels right now."

Move on to tapping point 3, the top of the head. Tap with all four fingers on both hands and say out loud:

"I love the way my body feels right now. I know my body responds this way to try to protect me. I know this is my body's natural reaction and I love and accept that my body wants me to be safe from harm. I am profoundly grateful for this reaction. I love and accept every part of my body and I love and accept all of the things it does for me."

Move on to tapping point 4, the eyebrows. You can tap on either side with two fingers. Switch sides when you go through the tapping sequence the second time. Say out loud as you tap:

"I know what it feels like to feel calm and free of stress. I know what it feels like to be completely safe, without any worries or disturbances in the world. I love and accept that my body wants to protect me from harm so that I may return to a peaceful calm. Even though I have so much anxiety and stress right now, I know what calm feels like."

Move on to tapping point 5, side of the eye. Tap with two fingers on either side. When you go through the tapping sequence the second time you can switch sides. Say out loud as you tap:

"I am open to feeling calm and relaxed as I move through my blockages and disturbances, releasing all of these intense emotions that have built up within me. Embracing calmness. Embracing peacefulness. Embracing my body's naturally peaceful flow of energy."

Move on to tapping point 6, under the eye. Tap with two fingers on either side. When you go through the tapping sequence the second time you can switch sides. Say out loud as you tap:

"I have control over my body. I have control over my emotions. I have control over all of my feelings. I have control over the way my energy flows. I am in control and no one else can control me. I can feel the stress and anxiety starting to leave my body. I can feel my energy starting to flow as the blockages and disturbances become smaller and smaller."

Move on to tapping point 7, under the nose. Tap with two fingers and say out loud as you tap:

"This remaining stress and intense emotions in my body are hard to let go of. I understand that my body does not want me to let it go. I understand that my body wants to keep it. My body wants to keep me safe. My body wants to protect me. And I've spent so much time trying to ignore it, or pretend it isn't there."

Move on to tapping point 8, the chin. Tap with two fingers and say out loud as you tap:

"But now I love and accept that my body responds this way. I profoundly love and accept myself, even with these overwhelming emotions. I profoundly love and accept every single part of myself even with all of this stress. And although I am now ready to let it go, I know that even if I don't let it go that I still completely love and accept every part of myself."

Move on to tapping point 9, the collarbone. You can tap on either side with all four fingers. Switch sides when you go through the tapping sequence the second time. Say out loud as you tap:

"But I am ready to let go of these remaining emotions that cause me turmoil. I do not need them anymore. I can feel them leaving my body and I can feel the calm and peace coming into my body. I know this feeling of peacefulness. I know this feeling of calm. And I embrace these feelings within me now."

Move on to tapping point 10, under your arm. Tap on either side with all four fingers. Switch sides when you go through the tapping sequence the second time. Say out loud as you tap:

"I may still feel stress, and I may still feel overwhelming emotions. I recognize it and I may feel it. But I will not criticize myself for having these feelings. I am choosing to just recognize that they are there and recognize how they feel. And it is OK. I love and accept myself even with all of these intense emotions. I love and accept that it is my body trying to protect me. And I love and accept myself enough to let it go."

If this was the first time you have tapped, congratulations! You have finished your first tapping session. Now that you have gone through it, ask yourself on a scale of 1 to 10 how are you feeling right now?

I've noticed with my clients that tapping through a general tapping sequence like this typically reduces their level of stress by at least 1 or 2 points each time through. You can go through the sequence again right now if you like, or you can continue reading and learn more about advanced tapping theory and practice so that future tapping sessions can be even more targeted, efficient, and effective. You can use tapping any time you feel stress, wherever you are, and as much as you want. That is one of the great things about tapping. You can do it by yourself, anywhere you are, whenever you feel you need it.

PART II: Advanced tapping: theory and practice

How EFT tapping affects the brain

We carry griefs, traumas and tensions with us all throughout our lives from our very earliest years. I am often asked about the root causes of problems we might experience in adulthood, such as post traumatic stress disorder, social phobia, or so other seemingly irrational fear or reaction. What happened in a person's life to make them this way? The answer is that often it is something devastating that occurred in childhood. It could be abuse that occurred, especially sexual abuse, and especially if the perpetrator was a trusted loved one like a parent or relative. It could be separation or a feeling of abandonment after a death or divorce.

Sometimes though, it is something else. For example, I recall a life coaching client I worked with years ago who recalled a story of his father happily throwing him in the air and catching him when he was a small child. They were both having great fun, until his father failed to catch him and he fell, striking the ground hard but sustaining only minor injuries. As no bones were broken, and whatever injuries he sustained quickly healed this didn't loom large in his memory has a major traumatic even in his childhood. Who would think such an event could have any effect on an adult, altering his character, his personality, and his life for decades? It is counter intuitive, but in fact when we tapped through this recollection it became clear to him in the days and weeks that followed that this seemingly small event was having a big impact on his personality.

What confuses this issue even further is the lack of consistency from person to person. We know from observing combat troops who have returned home after witnessing and participating in unspeakable horrors that not all of them have PTSD. Studies show that anywhere from 50% up to 75% actually do not suffer from PTSD, even after having completed one or more tours in combats like the Vietnam War, the Gulf War, the Iraq War, or the war in Afghanistan. Why is it that two troops stationed in the same location under the same commanding officer who carry out their duties together can return home together and only one of them suffers from PTSD? It is puzzling and intriguing and forces us to ask what exactly is it that triggers this severe trauma. For now, a full explanation of how this happens escapes all forms of modern medical science, healing, and wellness.

Although it would be interesting and probably useful to know how exactly how and why trauma effects people differently, what matters more is that we know how to deal with the trauma when we experience it. This is where tapping comes in. EFT tapping is, in a sense, a method for telling yourself over and over, in various ways, that you are safe. Notice that this is different from simply mentally reassuring ourselves that we are fine. When someone is feeling truly emotionally upset about something, the simple thought "don't worry" may not be very helpful.

What is more helpful is not just verbal reassurance, but also "pre-verbal" assurance and reassurance. The importance of pre-verbal communication is a consequence of the evolution of our human brains. Often times the part of our brains that most acutely perceives trauma signals from the body caused by emotional blockages are the more primitive or "reptilian" parts of the brain. These parts of the brain are located towards the back and the middle of the brain. As we developed into the intellectual, verbal, rational beings that we are today, our brains literally grew forwards. The most complex parts of our brains responsible for our highest order functions are thus directly behind our foreheads. As you go back further into the brain towards the back of the head, the processing power and ability becomes increasingly less logical and more reactionary. This is the part of the brain that dinosaurs had. It is the part of the brain that alligators have. The difference is that this is *all* they have. We have this older "reptilian" part of the brain, but then in addition we are fortunately endowed with all of our exceptional human critical faculties as well.

When you think of the things that are important to reptiles and animals living in the wild, you can get a sense of what this part of our human brain is responsible for. It is for surviving. It is for making quick, split-second decisions. Will this new thing I see/hear/experience hurt me? Do I fight? Do I flee? Am I hungry? Am I thirsty? Do I need to sleep? These basic functions are what this part of the brain is responsible for dealing with. Survival. What do I need to do to survive. That is it's only concern. It is unconcerned with language, complex reasoning, higher order wants or needs. All of these higher order concerns are left to the front parts of our brains.

Our "reptilian" brains thus preform a crucial function for us: they keep us safe. The downside however, is that they are not always very adept at dealing with modern society. They have a tendency to keep us *too* safe, by stoking up fears and panic, and trying to drive us away from anything it perceives to be dangerous even when the "danger" is actually no threat to our well-being, such as giving a speech in front of a large audience, asking someone you don't know well on a date, or dealing with lingering, subconscious memories of traumatic experiences that are now over.

Further, this oldest and most basic part of the brain is impervious to logic or language. Trying to tell this part of the brain "don't worry, everything is OK" is a bit like trying to reason with an alligator. It is not hearing or understanding you. It has no interest or ability to deal with such things.

The next part of the brain to develop is the middle part of the brain. This development occurred first with animals that are more advanced than reptiles. If you have a pet dog or cat, they have this middle part of the brain. We can actually perceive the difference when we look in the eye of an alligator or a lizard. There is nothing warm or emotionally responsive there. On the other hand, when we look a cat or dog in the eye, we sense that there is more going on there. There is the potential for some type of emotional relationship.

When trauma occurs, it can be recorded in the middle brain of an animal and subsequently activate the reptilian brain, triggering a survival response. This is something that has actually happened to most of us at some point (or more likely many points!) as we grew up. We experienced some kind of trauma, it was recorded in our middle brain, and when we experience certain similar stimulus in the future the middle brain triggers our reptilian brain to activate our "survival mode" response, even though the situation we are in doesn't really require it. This problem is further compounded when we lack the tools we need to communicate with the traumatized middle brain and the reactionary reptilian brain. Both of these parts of the brain are pre-verbal, so words alone won't work. The middle brain however is responsive to touch and certain sounds. This is why if your cat or dog is experiencing trauma, they will be responsive to gentle stroking, or soothing and calming voices. They will understand that this indicates there is no threat and that they can calm down and cease triggering a survival mode reaction in the reptilian brain.

EFT tapping is actually a similar tool for humans as stroking and soothing noises is for a cat or dog. It is a way of initiating a physiological communication with your body that tells it: "I'm safe. I'm OK. Everything is fine." The tapping that we do with EFT tells your body that there is no threat, there is no trauma, there is no need to activate our fight or flight survival mode response.

Reports from EFT practitioners who have dealt with veterans returning to the United States after serving in Iraq are highly encouraging. Some practitioners have suggested high rates of success in treating even high levels of PTSD after only a few tapping sessions. Many veterans in fact would go on to test negative on PTSD diagnostic tests after working with an EFT practitioner to tap through their trauma. Even the best of attempts to convince PTSD sufferers they are now safe and that the trauma is behind them have only moderate levels of success when they are aimed at appealing to the frontal brain (the verbal, rational, reasoning brain that exists directly behind our forehead). What happens if you introduce a bit of physical stimulation in the form of tapping though is remarkable. In doing this, you reach out to the middle brain, and in turn to the reptilian brain. The whole body becomes involved and the real healing can finally begin.

Targeting your tapping

In a nutshell, we tap in order to create a disruption within the mind-body communication. We want to alter our blockages and facilitate the proper flow of energy. But all the tapping in the world won't help to facilitate this proper flow of energy if you don't accurately target your tapping sessions. I've had people write to me, or I've met people in person at conferences who have shared with me that they've had mixed results with tapping. I ask them to take me through a typical tapping session as they would ordinarily do it themselves, and we discuss the tapping script they are using and what it is aimed at achieving. Often then begin with the usual "Even though I am ____" where the blank is filled with whatever difficulty they wish to overcome.

Let me share a particularly memorable encounter I had with a lady not that long ago who was somewhat new to EFT tapping. This lady suffered from sever Springtime allergies. She would practically sneeze and sniffle at the mere *thought* of Springtime. She was hopeful that she could harness the power of tapping to relieve her of these symptoms she had suffered from for years. I began by asking her to recall if there was a time in her life when she did not suffer from allergies in the Spring. I observed her as she started to think about my question and her body actually began to change, just in response to thinking about it. Allergies are sometimes not allergies at all, but rather they are adverse reactions caused by the unconscious which is responding to a disturbed emotional state somewhere within the body. In this lady's case, it was not the season of Spring that was causing her allergy. It was the her unconscious reaction that was causing her symptoms. We start tapping and I ask her what memories are coming up. She says she remembers her grandmother, and visiting her grandmother's big, old country home when she was a child. She said she must have been four or five years old and she dreaded visiting her grandmother. She told me that she hated her. Her grandmother was elderly and in a wheelchair and "mean as hell", she told me.

"When would you go to visit your grandmother?" I asked her.
"Every Spring when my dad would get his vacation from work," she told me. Her eyes opened wide with the realization of what she had just said.
I probed deeper as we continued to tap and the lady recalled that her grandmother would make her go outside and pull out the weeds from around her house using her bare hands. She would cut and chafe her hands on the weeds and cry and scream for her parents.

We tapped through her emotional blockages that had long been inhibiting her body's natural flow of energy. In her case, the blockages had ultimately manifested as an apparent allergy to Spring. The unconscious mind and an inhibited flow of energy can have strange and surprising consequences.

So, when you tap, what are you aiming at? You want to aim at what is inside. That could be emotions, it could be a picture, sound, smell, or it could be a sensation. I find it can be helpful to close my eyes and really try to focus on what my body is trying to tell me. Your body is constantly giving you feedback about what is right and what is wrong. The feedback can be subtle, but it is there if you are willing to take the time to really notice it. Listen to your body, think about your history and life experiences, especially as a child, and let your body guide your tapping to the right place.

Developing your own tapping scripts

As you gain more experience and comfort with using EFT tapping, you will eventually want to begin developing your own tapping scripts to use as a supplement to or as a replacement of the tapping scripts contained in this book or in other EFT resources you have consulted. This is a great way to move forward with your use of EFT tapping. In developing your own tapping scripts, there are certain features you will want to keep in mind. This section of the book aims to help you to develop your own tapping scripts, or improve on tapping scripts you have already created.

A very common mistake I see when people begin developing their own tapping scripts is that they will include a phrase that describes their problem as a concept distinct from its symptoms, rather than focusing on *their own subjective experience* of the problem. Recall that perhaps the most basic premise of EFT is that our problems are caused by disturbances in our energy field. The purpose of our tapping scripts therefore is to facilitate our physiological communication in such a way that we can remedy this disturbance through tapping. This means we need to be precise in choosing words that help us get in tune with the disturbance as accurately and as specifically as possible. We can do this by using words that describe our experience of the problem, rather than the general name or idea of the problem.

This description may be a bit abstract so let's work through some examples so you can see what I mean. Imagine it is almost time for you to give an important presentation at work and you can feel that you are beginning to sweat beneath your shirt. It may be tempting in this situation to begin a quick tapping sessions with the script

"Even though I am sweating, I deeply and profoundly love and accept myself..."

This may in the end be a helpful script, but it is less than ideal and your results could likely be improved by drilling down on your symptoms and really getting specific about them in your script. Simply saying "sweating" doesn't really capture how you experience the problem. The problem itself might be that you are feeling anxious, hot, and a little light-headed. The script could then become

"even though I am feeling anxious, hot, light-headed, and I'm sweating underneath my arms, I deeply and profoundly love and accept myself..."

At each point where you would have other wise just said "sweating" you would replace it with the much more specific "feeling anxious, hot, light-headed, and I'm sweating underneath my arms".

One of the general points you should keep in mind about developing tapping scripts is that you want to focus on emotions, or thoughts behind the emotions, rather than just physical sensations. These types of scripts help you to get at what the real problem actually is and can improve the efficiency and effectiveness of your tapping.

Here is another example: suppose that before leaving for work you had a dispute with your husband and left the house feeling angry at him. Here it is easy to name the feeling rather than a physical sensation. We can go deeper than this though. Rather than simply naming the emotion you are experiencing, you can get more specific by adding *why* you are experiencing the emotion. By including the reason you are experiencing the emotion instead of just stating the emotion itself you are again increasing the specificity and probably success of your tapping. Suppose that in this example you are angry at your husband because you felt he wasn't appreciative of some of the things things you have done around the house recently. Your tapping script might begin with something like this:

"Even though I am angry at my husband because he doesn't appreciate the fact that I am always the one who picks the kids up from school, I deeply and profoundly love and accept myself..."

We can go even further than this though. Once you've tapped on your specific script, you might start to ask yourself what the emotion or situation reminds you of. Maybe you remember feeling unappreciated as a child when you would look after your younger siblings and your parents would not appreciate how well you took care of them. Once you've identified this historic similarity, you could work the two experiences into your tapping script like this:

"Even though I am angry and hurt that my parents didn't appreciate how hard I tried to look after my younger siblings, and I am angry and hurt that my husband doesn't appreciate the fact that I always pick the kids up from school, I deeply and profoundly love and accept myself..."

This tapping phrase is digging even deeper, targeting not only the *emotion* and the *reason for the emotion*, but also the *historical source of the emotion*. Remember these strategies and apply them as you develop your own tapping scripts to boost your tapping efficiency and effectiveness!

Mindfulness

Mindfulness is being aware in the present moment. Too often our minds get caught up in the future, anticipating what might happen or dwelling on previous decisions that we regret. Virtually everyone spends too much time focusing on one or both of these areas and they do so at the expense of focusing on the present, the here and now. Mindfulness therefore is a meditative practice or method aimed at returning you to the present moment and appreciating everything that is going on in the present, both within you, and outside of you in the world.

Looking at a macro level, a mindful society is one that focuses on things like preventative health care and well-being, instead of just managing diseases once they've already occurred. It is teaching children how to be fully present in the moment, how to focus, how to complete the tasks assigned to them, rather than yelling at them for making excuses about not doing their homework.

Mindfulness can be transformational, for individuals and for all of us as a society. There is an increasing body of science backing up the importance of mindfulness as we continue to improve our understanding of how the brain works. It can benefit students and workers alike, preventing burn-out and stress from accumulating and ultimately contributing to ulcers, diabetes, heart disease, and so many other ailments that are caused by or contributed to by stress.

In some sense, we are all on a treadmill on our daily lives. Whether you are a construction worker, a retail cashier, an executive at a Fortune 500 company, or a single mother with two children, we are all on the treadmill. So how do we slow down and start appreciating life? What can we do to be more mindful in our daily lives?

One helpful method is to set a certain time every day or even just once a week, where you quietly reflect on the present. Where you are in your life. What you want. How you are feeling. It is best if you have a certain space where you can go for this ritual. It could be a room in your house or a bench at a local park. Wherever it is, it is your space and your time to be mindful and to shift your thoughts and perspective to the present. Turn your cell phone off and spend five minutes on this if that is all that you have. If you can take half an hour to do this. What matters most is not how long you spent being mindful per session, but rather than you do it regularly, ideally every day.

If you think of implementing a mindfulness schedule is too "out there" or "woo woo" first of all, realize that what we are talking about is simply focusing on yourself, regulating your breathing, and being in the moment. This is not some crazy new age religion that requires you to abandon whatever spiritual believes you are presently do or do not hold. Second of all, realize also that the United States Marine Core has implemented and continues to expand upon a mindfulness program to aid Marines in their clarity of thought and ability to live in the moment. This is true of many major companies nowadays as well, especially tech companies or those that deal in the "creative economy". These techniques are real. They work and are accepted by some of the least "woo woo" organizations you can imagine. So many people are currently benefiting from increasing their mindfulness and there is no reason that you shouldn't claim this benefit for yourself as well.

The coming paradigm shift

Even the most traditional and conservative members of the allopathic medical community accept that there are important connections between emotion and health, claiming that as much as 85% of all illnesses that manifest as physical problems are actually linked to a deeper emotional disturbance. Although many realize this, they often don't see the solution as being anything other than a prescription drug. This is very unfortunate and is probably a consequence of the pharmaceutical industry's aggressive lobbying of health care professionals. Much of modern medicine as essentially been "brainwashed" by the mantra that drugs must be used to treat all ailments, whether physical, psychological, or anything else.

EFT tapping seems to be very safe. There is virtually no opportunity to hurt someone with it, which cannot be said of most drug therapy. The only danger with EFT tapping, if there is one, is that its power and application could be miscommunicated. It would be unfortunate if anyone thought they could master EFT tapping in one session and that whatever results they had in that one sessions fully exhausted the power of EFT tapping. EFT tapping is easy to learn and apply as a beginner. This is one of it's many strengths. It is much more difficult to master however, and the more one studies and practices the application of EFT, the more effective their tapping sessions will become. The real danger is thus that one would fail to appreciate the true power of tapping and abandon it before seeing it's real potential.

EFT tapping is a truly amazing resource that belongs in everyone's "first aid" kit. There is perhaps no better tool for achieving your personal goals than regular application of EFT tapping. It is crucial however, that one understand the underlying source of negative thoughts, beliefs, and emotions, in order to get the full benefit from EFT tapping. We all have certain emotional blockages and negative beliefs. Many of them were installed by authority figures when we were younger, such as parents, teachers, older peers, religious leaders, etc. When one takes the time to appreciate and gain the insight into their emotional blockage, EFT tapping can be an amazingly powerful technique for clearing these blockages and positively transforming your life.

Perhaps the best example of something nearly everyone is dissatisfied with is their income level. This is an excellent example to work with because not only is it nearly universal but it can also be used to demonstrate an important principle: we must set "S.M.A.R.T." goals. That is, our goals must be specific, measurable, attainable, realistic, and time-oriented. If you set your goal this year as earning $1 million dollars but you are currently earning $20,000, you are probably not being realistic. A better approach might be to work in stages, aiming for a certain percentage increase consistently from year to year. Many people I have worked with have had profound success at growing their income significantly over time using this approach and tapping through their blockages and the things that have held them back from earning money in the past.

Early on in my research and exploration on EFT tapping, I discovered a common blockage that many people have about finances. Subconsciously, many people believe that they don't deserve to earn more than they already do. They feel unworthy, and although they may not be aware of this feeling, it exists and it holds them back. Realizing what emotional anchors are holding you back, and tapping through them, can lead to truly profound changes in your life.

While attending EFT tapping conferences I have been told by multiple doctors that they believe that virtually every severe autoimmune disease arises in part due to some type of emotional distress that occurred in the early years of the patients life and went unresolved in adulthood. This is huge. Some of the most crippling conditions humans can suffer from, such as multiple sclerosis and rheumatoid arthritis are autoimmune diseases. If the trend I have observed continues, the medical establishment may become increasingly aware of the power and utility of EFT tapping, and accepting of it's place at the cutting-edge of whole body wellness.

Some people I know who have benefited from EFT tapping have worked hard to research and understand exactly how and why it works from a scientific basis. Others don't concern themselves much with the scientific explanation and care only about the fact that it works well for them. Whatever camp you fall into, EFT tapping has the potential to radically transform your life in a positive way. Even the most informed and dedicated EFT researchers and practitioners don't have a full explanation of the power of EFT tapping. We understand and can explain some of it, while some of it still remains a mystery that we continue to attempt to unravel.

It is important to point out that EFT tapping alone cures nothing. What cures ailments and pathologies within the body is the body itself. Rather than being a self-contained cure, EFT tapping is more like a key that unlocks the physical, mental, and spiritual power of the body to purge itself of its problems and restore the natural flow of energy. Further, in our modern world, many of the most common and yet still intractable difficulties people suffer from are the result of lifestyle choices. Eating a poor diet, not getting enough exercise, smoking, drinking, etc, can all lead to debilitating disease and an early death. Harnessing the power of EFT tapping can empower anyone to commit to making better choices and to follow through on their commitments. Even people who have tried and failed at ever diet out there, or thought they could never quit smoking or go to the gym regularly have experienced success with EFT tapping.

Many people are skeptical of the power of what is ultimately a shockingly simple technique for wellness. How could something so simple work so well, they wonder? As I wrote previously in one of my earlier books, I too initially shared this skepticism. I just didn't see how EFT tapping could live up to the hype. I quickly became a believer however when I saw the positive changes in myself and in those around me that were brought about by EFT tapping. I now have the following advice for those who, like myself, may be skeptical about trying EFT tapping: hold your skepticism. I think the most helpful thing I can suggest is that even if you are not sure why or how, initially just believe that it works. I think that in life it is generally true that whatever you believe and consistently focus on an pay attention to you will attract into your life. If you go into each tapping session believing that this is a bunch of hogwash, and that it couldn't possibly have any real impact on your life, you may find that this is exactly your experience. But if you instead, approach EFT tapping with an open mind and an attitude of willing to give it a chance, you will likely find that it is the most amazing wellness tool you will ever encounter in your life.

I suspect that we may be at the beginning of a paradigm shift in our way of thinking. We are increasingly becoming aware of the fact that we are largely influenced and even "brainwashed" by the media. It is difficult to overcome beliefs that are consistently put to us by supposed experts in their fields. What people are starting to realize though is that there is a level of influence that exists "behind the scenes" that accounts for what experts are telling us. Due to factors and forces that are not always apparent, we can come to be told and ultimately believe in erroneous information. The solution to this, is to simply be open. Be open to new ideas and new possibilities. Understand that we are all humans and none of us has a perfect understanding of anything.

There are essentially two purposes to EFT tapping. One is to help people commit to the lifestyle changes they want to make, but haven't been able to. EFT tapping is a great tool for facilitating the emotional changes necessary to ultimately achieve one's goals. The other purpose is to address the direct emotional traumas people are experiencing that are leading to undesirable physiological changes within the body.

Affirmations

Affirmations are statements made out loud with the intention of establishing their truth. And here is a controversial claim I'd like to deal with in this chapter: Affirmations always work.

Yes, affirmations *always* work. Consider the following affirmation:

I am effortlessly physically fit and good looking right now.

Say this out loud to yourself. For virtually all of this, this is not true. Further, virtually all of us are well aware that this is not true. But say it out loud anyway. Try to make yourself believe it. The fact is that when we know what we are saying is a lie, there is a subconscious reaction to tack on an extra, unspoken addition to the end of our affirmation: a sarcastic *"yeah, right!"* or, *"no I'm not!"* or maybe even, *"bulls**t!"*. This unspoken addendum ends up being just as much a part of the affirmation as the spoken part. Regardless of the words that are coming out of our mouths when we affirm the example above, the true affirmation we are making is one that is actually consistent with our subconscious belief:

I am effortlessly physically fit and good looking right now... no I'm not!

That is the *real* affirmation we are making, and this is why I claim that affirmations always work. It is because the real affirmation includes that addition at the end, whether we say it out loud or not.

It is these snarky additions made by our self-conscious that are ripe for targeting with EFT Tapping. When that little voice somewhere deep in our subconscious casts aspersions or self-doubt on our vocalized affirmation, we can turn to tapping to eliminate it.

Let's work through this idea together. Think of a goal you might want to meet through EFT tapping. What would you like to do in your life that would be possible for you if only you could drop your emotional resistance. State it in a positive affirmation, like:

I will have no trouble meeting my goal of _____ .

Notice the self-talk that bubbles up from your self-conscious in response. For some of us it will be clear and demand our attention while for others it will be a slight and subtle nagging lurking below the surface of our attention. Regardless of how forcefully our subconscious presents the addendum to the affirmation it is a powerful part of our believes and commitment to following through on the affirmation. Maybe your affirmation is that you want to double your income.

"I will have no trouble meeting my goal of doubling my income." To which your subconscious might add: *"but I've never done that before!"* Or: *"That will never work!"*

You might think of this subconscious nagging as the classic demon sitting on your shoulder, trying to bring you down. The fact though, is that it is not trying to bring you down. In fact, it is not a malicious demon at all. The subconscious reply is one that is designed to keep you safe. It is perfectly normal and natural response born out of our biological "fight or flight" impulse. When we face a challenging situation, our body naturally wants to keep us safe. In the wild, this often meant fleeing from the situation as the challenges that primitive man faced were often ones that could kill him, like a tiger lurking behind a bush waiting for its next meal. This is why the tapping scripts I use and the ones contained in this book express an appreciation for these types of seemingly self-destructive reactions. In fact, we need to be thankful for these reactions. We tap on them and express our gratitude. We appreciate them, rather than suppress them, or be upset by them, for contradicting our affirmations.

When you vocalize an affirmation that you don't fully believe in, such as in the example I gave above, every part of your psyche that disagrees will demand attention. It may do so subtly, or it may do so powerfully, but one way or another that part of your psyche will demand and receive attention, even if it is at the subconscious level.

What often happens is that when you deliberately focus your attention on one of these parts of your psyche that disagrees with your affirmation, the other parts become increasingly demanding of attention as well. It is easy to jump from focusing on one critical inner voice, to another, to another, to another, until before we know it we are in a spiral of negativity that while well-intentioned, serves to hold us back from taking action to achieve our goals.

This is what we must tap on. These negative addendums to our affirmations that are holding us back. Continuing with the example above, we would include in our tapping script something like:

I am thankful that my body tells me I am not effortlessly physically fit and good looking right now. I appreciate and am grateful that my body wants to keep me safe. Thank you, for helping me all this time. But I am a grown and mature adult now, and I can commit to my own goals and follow through completely with every part of my mind, body, and spirit.

EFT and positivity

I've presented and attended numerous conferences on EFT tapping and other facets of energy psychology over the years and it has happened a few times that I've been asked a particular question: Why is EFT tapping so focused on negativity? Why is it that people are so often tapping on getting rid of the negative aspects of their lives, rather than building the positive ones?

This is a very legitimate question based on a keen observation of EFT tapping sessions. We so often tap on what is bringing us down in order to release the negative charge of those emotions. We tap to eliminate pain and suffering from our lives, to deal with our financial or relationship problems, to lose weight or eliminate other ailments from our live. It may seem that we as EFT trainers and practitioners are dwelling on the negative at the expense of the positive. Why do we do this?

The answer is not that we like to dwell on what is negative. Rather, the reason why we so often deal with negative emotions is that EFT tapping cannot be effective when it is used to attempt to install positive emotions, beliefs, and affirmations on top of a foundation of contradictory negative beliefs. To do so would be like building the beautiful mansion of your dreams on top of a bed of quicksand. The reality is that no matter how often you state that you are perfectly happy, emotionally at peace, or ready for any challenge, if there are parts of you that don't believe it those parts will ultimately drag you down.

You may say in your affirmation:

"I am perfect, whole, and complete!"

But if your subconscious addendum is:

"actually, I'm a wreck!"

Then you will never get anywhere until you properly identify and tap through the unspoken addendum to your affirmation. It is essential that we take the time to deal with these underlying criticisms and self-doubt before we expect to make any long-term progress on our goals. We need a solid foundation before we can build our house. If you try to just say the positive affirmation without dealing with everything else below you are merely skinning the ulcer, rather than cutting it out.

It is a consequence of being raised in modern society that we naturally want to do the opposite of what we need to do to deal with negative thoughts and feelings. Think of conflicts you may have with coworkers or family members, for example. We are often taught as children to turn the other cheek in the fact of conflict. To not make a scene. To smile and put on a happy face, regardless of how you are really feeling. While this attitude may provide a necessary lubricant in certain interpersonal relationships, it is a dangerous attitude to apply to the relationship we have with ourselves and the interactions between the various parts of our bodies, minds, and spirits.

We must not ignore the doubt, hurt, or pain that lurks inside us. We must identify it, appreciate it, and tap on it. Only through this process can we reach a solid foundation and begin confidently stating our positive affirmations, knowing that our whole body is saying *"Yes! Yes! That's right! I can do it!"*.

Chakra clearing

In this chapter we will discuss the importance of regularly clearing out the whole system by using an exercise called "chakra clearing". This is a great exercise to do daily if you have the self-discipline, or once in awhile after a particularly intense tapping session.

Sometimes when employing EFT Tapping to deal with strong emotions we are left feeling "out of it" or suffering from a mental fogginess or lack of clarity. This is a good sign: it means we have made significant progress in dealing with our troubles. When we are left with this foggy feeling it is often due to the chakra centers being clogged. The chakras are important to our overall feeling of well-being because they are the centers where energy is stored. You might think of them as a sort of "intersection" for the body's energy. When the traffic lights are working and the traffic is not too heavy, everything will flow smoothly as it is meant to. But if the traffic lights malfunction, there is an accident, some construction on the road, or the traffic is just abnormally heavy, chaos and even gridlock can ensue. There is numerous analogies that can be made here. Think of traffic light failure as a physical shutdown of some of the bodies systems caused by excessive stress, caused for example by money or relationship problems. Think of a traffic accident as a collision between powerful but incompatible emotions, such as the exhilaration of getting a big promotion accompanied by fear and self-doubt that you can actually handle the increased responsibilities. And finally, think of increased traffic flow as the consequence of a vigorous tapping session, where energy and emotions are flowing through the system with greater intensity than usual. In all of these cases, we can facilitate a return to our natural and proper energy flow by clearing the chakras.

This exercise targets five of the body's chakras for clearing. When you first begin using the chakra clearing exercise below, I recommend that you go through each and every one of the five chakras in the order that is presented. This will give you the best chance of clearing out your chakras and restoring the body's natural flow of energy with one or two sessions of this exercise. When you become more experienced in clearing your chakras, you may find that you can identify which chakra or chakras need clearing before beginning the exercise, and then you will be able to focus only on those chakras that need clearing while ignoring the rest that are flowing normally. In my experience, the first two or three chakras that are covered in this exercise become blocked and in need of clearing more than the other chakras. All of the chakras are important, however. If any one of them is blocked it can cause serious emotional and physical distress that can lead to a variety of unpleasant acute or even chronic conditions. Until you become more comfortable with clearing your chakras, it is best to complete the entire exercise without skipping any chakras.

Chakra clearing exercise introduction

Let's begin the exercise. This exercise is a reliable way to clear the chakras and restore the natural flow of energy to the body and its systems. I caution you though that it is a bit more of an advanced technique and it can take awhile to get all the points down, especially if you want to use a script while tapping to clear the chakras. Don't expect perfection on your first time through. It is an exercise you can improve at as you get more comfortable with it, and especially as you become more in tune with the feedback you are getting from your body.

As always, get in a comfortable position. You could sit in a chair if you like, or on the floor. If you choose to sit on the floor, make sure you keep your back straight throughout the exercise. It may be helpful if you sit against a wall or other flat object. You can stand too if you prefer. Once you're in a comfortable position, take a moment to appreciate the feelings running through your body. Whatever it is that you are feeling, rate it out of 10. For example if you are feeling stressed, rate it out of 10, where 1 is very little or no stress, up to 10 being maximum stress.

Start the exercise by tapping each pair of fingers together, one pair at a time. Start with the tips of the thumbs first and tap them together ten times. Next, tap the tips of the forefingers together ten times. Then the middle fingers, the ring fingers, and little fingers, tapping ten times each, one pair at a time.

Next, rub the hands together briskly, moving them in a circular motion about 15 times as you begin to focus your thoughts entirely on the body, ignoring as best you can any external noise or distractions.

Crown chakra

Place an open hand, palm down, directly on the crown of your head. Start with your dominant hand. Do not place it to the front, the back, or either side. Place the palm directly on the center. Imagine there is a straight pole running up through your body. Place the palm of your hand at the top of the pole. Notice the feelings you are experiencing as you hold your palm on the crown of your head. Notice the subtle feelings going on inside your body. This can take focus and practice. Notice things like how tired you feel. Does your body feel heavy or light? Do you feel energetic? Stressed? Excited? Angry? Insecure? Anxious? Take a few moments until you feel you have a grasp of these feelings as they currently exist inside the body.

Next, begin tapping through the following tapping points using the other hand. Tap on each point for 10 to 20 seconds. As you tap through the points, focus your attention on the hand that is on the crown of your head. Breathe in and out, slowly and deeply, as you continue to tap through all of the following tapping points while maintaining your focus on the hand on top of your head.

Start with the inside of the eyebrow, and as you tap, continue to focus your attention on the hand on top of your head.

Tap at the side of the eye, still focusing on the other hand and breathing in and out in a slow and controlled manner.

Tap underneath the eye at the cheekbone.

Next, move to the inside of the other eyebrow, and then to the side of that eye, tapping and continuing to focus on the hand on your head.

Tap under your nose. Focus only on the hand on the top of your head, still controlling your breathing.

Next, tap under your mouth. Focus on the hand on the top of your head. Take a deep breath in and out.

Next, tap your collarbone as you continue focusing on the other hand and breathing in and out in a slow and controlled manner.

Now, use your index finger to tap on the normal tapping point on the outer side of the thumb. If you have someone with you, you could have them do the tapping for you. If not, you can do it on your own instead. Maintain your focus on the hand that is on top of your head. Continue breathing slowly, in and out.

Use your thumb to tap the point on the side of your index finger, still focusing your attention on the hand on the crown of your head.

Next, use your thumb to tap the side of your middle finger. Focus only on the hand on the top of your head. Take a deep breath in and out.

Now tap your ring finger, still using your thumb. Focus your attention on the hand on the crown of your head as you breathe slowly, in and out.

Finally, tap your little finger with your thumb as you continue breathing slowly, in and out, still focusing on the hand on top of your head.

Put both your hands at your sides and take a moment now to notice how you feel. Do you feel more relaxed? Less stressed? Less anxious? How would you rate your current emotional state out of 10? Is it better than when we began this exercise? Maybe you are already noticing a change. If so, that is great, but it is OK if you're not.

Third eye chakra

Let's move onto the "third eye" chakra. Put the palm of your dominant hand directly over the point in between your two eyebrows. Make sure the center of the palm is over the point, not the wrist, or fingers.

Start by tapping at the side of the eye, focusing on the other hand over your third eye and breathing in and out in a slow and controlled manner.

Tap underneath the same eye at the cheekbone.

Next, move to the side of the other eye, tapping and continuing to focus on the other hand over your third eye.

Tap under your nose. Focus only on the hand on the over your third eye, still controlling your breathing.

Next, tap under your mouth. Focus on the hand on the over your third eye. Take a deep breath in and out.

Next, tap your collarbone as you continue focusing on the other hand and breathing in and out in a slow and controlled manner.

Now, use your index finger to tap on the normal tapping point on the outer side of the thumb. If you have someone with you, you could have them do the tapping for you. If not, you can do it on your own instead. Maintain your focus on the hand that is over your third eye . Continue breathing slowly, in and out.

Use your thumb to tap the point on the side of your index finger, still focusing your attention on the hand over your third eye.

Next, use your thumb to tap the side of your middle finger. Focus only on the hand over your third eye. Take a deep breath in and out.

Now tap your ring finger, still using your thumb. Focus your attention on the hand over your third eye as you breathe slowly, in and out.

Finally, tap your little finger with your thumb as you continue breathing slowly, in and out, still focusing on the hand over your third eye.

Put both your hands at your sides and take a moment now to notice how you feel. Many people notice a big difference at this point. How do you feel? Do you feel more relaxed? Less stressed? Less anxious? How would you rate your current emotional state out of 10? Is it better than when we began this exercise? If there is no change, it's OK. Persevere through the exercise and clearing the other chakras, or return to the exercise later when you are more in tune with your body.

Neck chakra

Now let's move on to the chakra in the neck/throat. Put the center of the palm of your dominant hand over your throat. If you are a man, this is where your Adam's apple is. If you are a woman, look straight ahead and position your hand such that the side of the index finger is resting underneath your chin.

Next, begin tapping through the following tapping points using the other hand. As you tap through the points, focus your attention on the hand that is over your throat. Breathe in and out, slowly and deeply, as you continue to tap through all of the following tapping points while maintaining your focus on the hand over your throat.

Start with the inside of the eyebrow, and as you tap, continue to focus your attention on the hand over your throat.

Tap at the side of the eye, still focusing on the other hand and breathing in and out in a slow and controlled manner.

Tap underneath the eye at the cheekbone.

Next, move to the inside of the other eyebrow, and then to the side of that eye, tapping and continuing to focus on the hand over your throat.

Tap under your nose. Focus only on the hand over your throat, still controlling your breathing.

Next, tap under your mouth. Focus on the hand over your throat. Take a deep breath in and out.

Next, tap your collarbone as you continue focusing on the other hand and breathing in and out in a slow and controlled manner.

Now, use your index finger to tap on the normal tapping point on the outer side of the thumb. If you have someone with you, you could have them do the tapping for you. If not, you can do it on your own instead. Maintain your focus on the hand that is over your throat. Continue breathing slowly, in and out.

Use your thumb to tap the point on the side of your index finger, still focusing your attention on the hand over your throat.

Next, use your thumb to tap the side of your middle finger. Focus only on the hand over your throat. Take a deep breath in and out.

Now tap your ring finger, still using your thumb. Focus your attention on the hand over your throat as you breathe slowly, in and out.

Finally, tap your little finger with your thumb as you continue breathing slowly, in and out, still focusing on the hand over your throat.

Put both your hands at your sides and take a moment now to notice how you feel. Do you feel more relaxed? Less stressed? Less anxious? How would you rate your current emotional state out of 10? Is it better than when we began this exercise?

Solar plexus chakra

The next chakra is about two inches lower than the chakra we just cleared in the neck/throat, and is even with where your collarbones would meet in the center of your chest. Put the center of the palm of your dominant hand over that point. This chakra is sometimes refereed to as the "solar plexus" chakra.

Next, begin tapping through the following tapping points using the other hand. As you tap through the points, focus your attention on the hand that is over the "solar plexus" chakra. Breathe in and out, slowly and deeply, as you continue to tap through all of the following tapping points while maintaining your focus on the hand over the "solar plexus" chakra.

Start with the inside of the eyebrow, and as you tap, continue to focus your attention on the hand over the "solar plexus" chakra.

Tap at the side of the eye, still focusing on the other hand over the "solar plexus" chakra and breathing in and out in a slow and controlled manner.

Tap underneath the eye at the cheekbone while focusing on the hand over the "solar plexus" chakra.

Next, move to the inside of the other eyebrow, and then to the side of that eye, tapping and continuing to focus on the hand over the "solar plexus" chakra.

Tap under your nose. Focus only on the hand over the "solar plexus" chakra, still controlling your breathing.

Next, tap under your mouth. Focus on the hand over the "solar plexus" chakra. Take a deep breath in and out.

Next, tap your collarbone as you continue focusing on the other hand and breathing in and out in a slow and controlled manner.

Now, use your index finger to tap on the normal tapping point on the outer side of the thumb. If you have someone with you, you could have them do the tapping for you. If not, you can do it on your own instead. Maintain your focus on the hand that is over the "solar plexus" chakra. Continue breathing slowly, in and out.

Use your thumb to tap the point on the side of your index finger, still focusing your attention on the hand over the "solar plexus" chakra.

Next, use your thumb to tap the side of your middle finger. Focus only on the hand over the "solar plexus" chakra. Take a deep breath in and out.

Now tap your ring finger, still using your thumb. Focus your attention on the hand over the "solar plexus" chakra as you breathe slowly, in and out.

Finally, tap your little finger with your thumb as you continue breathing slowly, in and out, still focusing on the hand over the "solar plexus" chakra.

Put both your hands at your sides and take a moment now to notice how you feel. Do you feel more relaxed? Less stressed? Less anxious? How would you rate your current emotional state out of 10? Is it better than when we began this exercise?

Below the belly button chakra

Place the palm of your dominant hand one inch below your belly button. Breathe in and out, slowly and deeply, as you continue to tap through all of the following tapping points while maintaining your focus on the hand one inch below your belly button.

Start with the inside of the eyebrow, and as you tap, continue to focus your attention on the hand one inch below your belly button.

Tap at the side of the eye, still focusing on the other hand and breathing in and out in a slow and controlled manner.

Tap underneath the eye at the cheekbone.

Next, move to the inside of the other eyebrow, and then to the side of that eye, tapping and continuing to focus on the hand one inch below your belly button.

Tap under your nose. Focus only on the hand on the top of your head, still controlling your breathing.

Next, tap under your mouth. Focus on the hand one inch below your belly button. Take a deep breath in and out.

Next, tap your collarbone as you continue focusing on the other hand and breathing in and out in a slow and controlled manner.

Now, use your index finger to tap on the normal tapping point on the outer side of the thumb. Continue breathing slowly, in and out.

Use your thumb to tap the point on the side of your index finger, still focusing your attention on the hand one inch below your belly button.

Next, use your thumb to tap the side of your middle finger. Focus only on the hand one inch below your belly button. Take a deep breath in and out.

Now tap your ring finger, still using your thumb. Focus your attention on the hand one inch below your belly button as you breathe slowly, in and out.

Finally, tap your little finger with your thumb as you continue breathing slowly, in and out, still focusing on the hand one inch below your belly button.

Put both your hands at your sides and take a moment now to notice how you feel. Do you feel more relaxed? Less stressed? Less anxious? Maybe you are already notice a change. If so, that is great, but it is OK if you're not.

Further chakra clearing

If you have made it through the entire exercise and have not noticed an improvement there are two options: (1) Go through each chakra again, this time switching hands so that you are using your weaker hand to cover the chakras and your dominant hand to tap. (2) Come back to this exercise later when you are feeling more in tune with your body.

This exercise may not be helpful every time you do it. If you are experience a different emotional problem unrelated to blocked chakras or if you are simply not sufficiently in tune with your body's feedback, you may find you get little out of this exercise. More often, however, I find that this exercise can make a significant difference in a person's disposition, bringing them down several points on the ten point scale. Also, remember that as you become more experienced at using this exercise, you will be able to target and clear the chakras with greater accuracy and efficiency. I understand it is a long exercise initially, but as with so many things in life, rewards come to those who persevere.

The first few times through the chakra clearing exercise you may find it difficult to work with a script while tapping. There are many spots to remember to tap and I'm sure you will need to refer to this book as you go through the exercise. That is fine. As you become more advanced at clearing the chakras and you need to refer less and less to the instructions in this chapter, you can begin to incorporate a script into the chakra clearing exercise, just as you would use a script as part of a tapping sequence. I'd encourage you to use the instructions contained in this book in the chapters on targeting your tapping and developing your own tapping script to customize your own script to use during this exercise. In case you need some help getting started though, I'll include below a general chakra clearing script and instructions on how to clear the crown chakra as you are using it. I hope you find it helpful.

Crown chakra clearing script

As explained above, place an open hand, palm down, directly on the crown of your head. Start with your dominant hand. Do not place it to the front, the back, or either side. Place the palm directly on the center. Imagine there is a straight pole running up through your body. Place the palm of your hand at the top of the pole. Notice the feelings you are experiencing as you hold your palm on the crown of your head. Notice the subtle feelings going on inside your body. This can take focus and practice. Notice things like how tired you feel. Does your body feel heavy or light? Do you feel energetic? Stressed? Excited? Angry? Insecure? Anxious? Take a few moments until you feel you have a grasp of these feelings as they currently exist inside the body.

Next, begin tapping through the following tapping points using the other hand. Tap on each point for 10 to 20 seconds. As you tap through the points, focus your attention on the hand that is on the crown of your head. Breathe in and out, slowly and deeply, as you continue to tap through all of the following tapping points while maintaining your focus on the hand on top of your head.

Start with the inside of the eyebrow, and as you tap, continue to focus your attention on the hand on top of your head. Say out loud:

"even though I am feeling so much stress, and overwhelming emotions right now, I profoundly and completely love and accept myself. I profoundly love and accept the way I feel right now. I profoundly love and accept myself and everything that I am."

Tap at the side of the eye, still focusing on the other hand and breathing in and out in a slow and controlled manner.

"Even though I feel so much stress and turmoil in my life right now. Even though sometimes the stress feels overwhelming. Even though sometimes I feel like I can't focus on anything or function the way I want to because of these intense feelings. Even though I feel this way, I profoundly love and accept myself, and my body, and the way it feels right now."

Tap underneath the eye at the cheekbone.

"I love the way my body feels right now. I know my body responds this way to try to protect me. I know this is my body's natural reaction and I love and accept that my body wants me to be safe from harm. I am profoundly grateful for this reaction. I love and accept every part of my body and I love and accept all of the things it does for me."

Next, move to the inside of the other eyebrow, and then to the side of that eye, tapping and continuing to focus on the hand on your head.

"I know what it feels like to feel calm and free of stress. I know what it feels like to be completely safe, without any worries or disturbances in the world. I love and accept that my body wants to protect me from harm so that I may return to a peaceful calm. Even though I have so much anxiety and stress right now, I know what calm feels like."

Tap under your nose. Focus only on the hand on the top of your head, still controlling your breathing.

"I am open to feeling calm and relaxed as I move through my blockages and disturbances, releasing all of these intense emotions that have built up within me. Embracing calmness. Embracing peacefulness. Embracing my body's naturally peaceful flow of energy."

Next, tap under your mouth. Focus on the hand on the top of your head. Take a deep breath in and out.

"I have control over my body. I have control over my emotions. I have control over all of my feelings. I have control over the way my energy flows. I am in control and no one else can control me. I can feel the stress and anxiety starting to leave my body. I can feel my energy starting to flow as the blockages and disturbances become smaller and smaller."

Next, tap your collarbone as you continue focusing on the other hand and breathing in and out in a slow and controlled manner.

"This remaining stress and intense emotions in my body are hard to let go of. I understand that my body does not want me to let it go. I understand that my body wants to keep it. My body wants to keep me safe. My body wants to protect me. And I've spent so much time trying to ignore it, or pretend it isn't there."

Now, use your index finger to tap on the normal tapping point on the outer side of the thumb. If you have someone with you, you could have them do the tapping for you. If not, you can do it on your own instead. Maintain your focus on the hand that is on top of your head. Continue breathing slowly, in and out.

"But now I love and accept that my body responds this way. I profoundly love and accept myself, even with these overwhelming emotions. I profoundly love and accept every single part of myself even with all of this stress. And although I am now ready to let it go, I know that even if I don't let it go that I still completely love and accept every part of myself."

Use your thumb to tap the point on the side of your index finger, still focusing your attention on the hand on the crown of your head.

"But I am ready to let go of these remaining emotions that cause me turmoil. I do not need them anymore. I can feel them leaving my body and I can feel the calm and peace coming into my body."

Next, use your thumb to tap the side of your middle finger. Focus only on the hand on the top of your head. Take a deep breath in and out.

"I know this feeling of peacefulness. I know this feeling of calm. And I embrace these feelings within me now."

Now tap your ring finger, still using your thumb. Focus your attention on the hand on the crown of your head as you breathe slowly, in and out.

"I may still feel stress, and I may still feel overwhelming emotions. I recognize it and I may feel it. But I will not criticize myself for having these feelings. I am choosing to just recognize that they are there and recognize how they feel. And it is OK."

Finally, tap your little finger with your thumb as you continue breathing slowly, in and out, still focusing on the hand on top of your head.

I love and accept myself even with all of these intense emotions. I love and accept that it is my body trying to protect me. And I love and accept myself enough to let it go."

Put both your hands at your sides and take a moment now to notice how you feel. Do you feel more relaxed? Less stressed? Less anxious? How would you rate your current emotional state out of 10? Is it better than when we began this exercise? Maybe you are already noticing a change. If so, that is great, if not proceed to clear the next chakra.

Blaming others to escape personal responsibility

We have all experienced some kind of trauma at various points in our lives. Sometimes, this trauma becomes connected to things we may have been thinking about at the time, or things that existed in our subconscious mind at time that was contemporaneous with the experience of trauma. Further, we have all experienced hypnosis at various points in our lives. Hypnosis is not something associated exclusively with the classic example of watching a pocket watch swing from one side to another and becoming drowsy. Indeed, it is highly debatable whether hypnosis can be induced this way at all. In any even, the concept of hypnosis is much broader than this. Hypnosis is your mind's ability to generate and imagine sensations and feelings of something that does not presently exist. Humans actually do this naturally and frequently. In some sense, we are frequently "living in the past". And when we live in the past, we feel emotions and experience reactions that are connected to some memory from long ago. The brain communicates these emotions to the body and the body in turn communicates it's reaction to the brain. In this way, hypnosis is a circle of life-like feedback loop that circulates through the body and drives us back to certain moments in our past. While the moment itself often escapes our conscious awareness, the associated feelings flood our consciousness and are just as real as if they were triggered by a present event.

There are some individuals who try tapping a few times and then stop. Maybe they use it to clear a particular blockage and then stop as soon as they think they've been successful in doing so. They think they are cured. But when people try tapping a few times and then stop, they often revert back to the problem they were having before. This is because growth and healing is a continual process. It is not the sort of thing that can be done once and then forgotten about. Either you focus on healing for your whole life, or you will tend to become increasingly unwell throughout your life instead. This is because without a clear path to wellness and positivity like the one tapping provides, you will start manifesting, and practicing, and focusing, on the negative aspects of your life. In order to break out of this, you need to do something differently.

You may be trying the same things over and over again, trying to improve your life but feeling like you are just running on a treadmill and getting nowhere. They wonder why their lives are still a mess. The answer is because they keep making the same mistakes over and over again. Imagine going to the doctor and telling him how your head hurts because you bumped it on a wall. And imagine further, the doctor telling you to go ahead and bump it on the wall again and see if you feel better. You won't feel better of course, you'll feel worse. This is what happens when you keep practicing the things you don't want. The results just get worse.

For some people there is a price to doing this. The price is throwing away the excuses that shield them from responsibility. It means not blaming your own difficult upbringing when you lose your temper with your own children. It means not justifying your inability to truly commit to a relationship because you were hurt in the past. It means not blaming the economy, the government, or society for your own unwillingness to work hard at a job or in school. I want to be clear that not everyone clings to excuses like these, but enough people do that it is worth mentioning here. It is also worth mentioning that lots of people who do this initially deny it. Take a moment and consider, as honestly and openly as you can, whether you are ever inclined to make excuses and blame your own shortcoming on something else. If you are doing this, you need to recognize that you are doing it before you can commit to abandoning this destructive practice.

When you heal yourself on the inside, and when you truly come to love and care about yourself, and when you learn to forgive those who have harmed you in the past, you begin the true journey of healing.

If you suspect you may be clinging to excuses that are interfering with your ability to live the best life possible, a good exercise is to start what I call a "positive journal". This is simply a journal that you use to record the positive, good, happy things that have happened to you or that you made happen. It is best when you write in the journal at least once a day, perhaps before you go to bed at night. Record your positive memories, positive emotional states, or anything that you think is uplifting. Then when you are having a bad day you can flip open the journal, think of the good things, and take personal accountability for your feelings. Realize that no one has more power to influence your well being than you do yourself. It is a powerful exercise.

Speaking personally, I know that some years ago before I discovered EFT tapping I was facing some challenging personal problems. They felt overwhelming at times. I am ashamed to admit that too often I would blame other people for the problems I was experiencing. I would blame family, friends, acquaintances, politicians, anyone I could think of. Today, I don't blame anyone. I accept responsibility and accountability for myself and I look for opportunities to grow as a human being. If you find yourself blaming others for your problems or dwelling on past events as the reason why you can't succeed in the future, you are on the wrong path. You are carrying around a sack of rotten memories and resentments that are weighing you down. You need to drop this sack by committing to not making excuses or blaming others. Think of all that you have to be thankful for, and start writing in your positive journal daily.

Why isn't EFT tapping working for me?

I can say that in my experience, EFT tapping works for virtually every single person I have ever encountered *when it is applied in the correct way*. It is possible however to apply the EFT tapping techniques incorrectly. When done incorrectly, EFT tapping may not work very well or indeed, it may not work at all. The key to success with EFT tapping is applying the methods correctly and consistently as part of your regular wellness routine.

If you have tried tapping through your problems and are not experiencing any progress, there are three main reasons why this might be happening.

One reason is that you may have a particular resistance to letting go of the energy blockage that is the source of your problem. The second reason is that you might not be targeting your tapping correctly and accurately. For example you may be using a poorly crafted tapping script or you might be tapping on the wrong points. The third reason is that there may be a pre-existing memory that is preventing you from clearing the blockage. I will describe each of these potential problems in detail in the hopes that this might help you to trouble-shoot your tapping and experience the same success so many others have had with this technique.

Resistance

When you are seeking to overcome a problem you are experiencing in your life, for example an undue amount of stress in your life, you may become very excited by the prospect. This is natural. Thinking about putting our problems behind us and moving on from them no longer encumbered by their weight is naturally a very exciting prospect. There is also, however, a natural tendency to worry about performing adequately once the problem is resolved. If you have feel you have been held back by stress and you believe that you can move forward in life and achieve your goals once you resolve your high stress level, you may feel once your stress problems are resolved you will no longer have an excuse for not achieving the things you want in your life. Essentially, your excuse will be gone and a failure will not be the fault of stress but rather it will be your fault and your fault alone. Perversely, this can actually induce stress in itself! You are in a sense seeking to cut a safety net that you may have been relying on to some extent as an excuse for the failure in your life or for not achieving your goals. This means that while one part of you is excited and looking forward to the future, the other is cowering in fear, clinging to the familiar rather than braving the unknown. This is a problem that must be addressed.

Letting go of this problem could be simple. It could be as simple as letting go of a particular bothersome or shameful memory. Tapping directly on that shameful experience or memory, if you are able to identify it, can be a quick solution for some people.

Another potential solution is to identify and acknowledge the resistance that you are experiencing and tap directly on the resistance. The way you would do this is by crafting a tapping script that states something like the following. As always, begin by assessing your issue, in this case your resistance, on a scale of 1 to 10.

If you would benefit from a visual aid as you proceed through this tapping sequence, remember that I have prepared a free video demonstration for readers of this book. If you think this would be helpful for you, please visit my website at **www.randallawrence.com** to get access to this free video and use it to help you tap through this sequence.

Start by tapping with four fingers on point 1, the side of the hand (or the "karate chop point"). Tap gently. There is no need to be aggressive with yourself or hurt yourself. Say out loud:

"Even though my body is resisting my attempts to clear my blockages [or distress, or whatever your specific issue is], I profoundly and completely love and accept myself. I profoundly love and accept the way I feel right now. I profoundly love and accept myself and everything that I am."

Move on to tapping on point 2, the inner wrist. You can tap with two fingers, four fingers, or your opposite wrist. Say out loud:

"Even though I am experiencing resistance in achieving the things I want to achieve. Even though this resistance can seem overwhelming. Even though sometimes I feel like I can't ever let go of this resistance. Even though I feel this way, I profoundly love and accept myself, and my body, and the way it feels right now."

Move on to tapping point 3, the top of the head. Tap with all four fingers on both hands and say out loud:

"I profoundly love and accept that my body is only trying to protect me from harm. I appreciate that it can be difficult and frightening to clear my blockages and overcome my challenges. But I will be brave. I will be brave and I will let go of the things that hold me back. I am ready to let go of the things that are holding me back. I have the courage to move forward in life and I will love and accept myself regardless of the outcome."

Move on to tapping point 4, the eyebrows. You can tap on either side with two fingers. Switch sides when you go through the tapping sequence the second time. Say out loud as you tap:

"I know what it feels like to let go of this resistance. I know what it feels like to be completely unencumbered. I know what it feels like not to be held back. I love and accept that my body wants to protect me from harm so that I may return to a peaceful calm. Even though my body is resisting my attempts to clear my blockages right now, I know what it feels like to let go."

Move on to tapping point 5, side of the eye. Tap with two fingers on either side. When you go through the tapping sequence the second time you can switch sides. Say out loud as you tap:

"I am open to letting go of my blockages and disturbances, moving forward, and embracing a life with stress [or whatever your specific issue is]. Embracing peacefulness. Embracing my body's naturally peaceful flow of energy."

Move on to tapping point 6, under the eye. Tap with two fingers on either side. When you go through the tapping sequence the second time you can switch sides. Say out loud as you tap:

"I have control over my body. I have control over my emotions. I have control over all of my feelings. I have control over the way my energy flows. I am in control and no one else can control me. I can feel resistance beginning to fade. I can feel my energy starting to flow as the blockages and disturbances become smaller and smaller."

Move on to tapping point 7, under the nose. Tap with two fingers and say out loud as you tap:

"This remaining resistance in my body is hard to let go of. I understand that my body does not want me to let it go. I understand that my body wants to keep it. My body wants to keep me safe. My body wants to protect me. And I've spent so much time trying to ignore it, or pretend it isn't there."

Move on to tapping point 8, the chin. Tap with two fingers and say out loud as you tap:

"But now I love and accept that my body responds this way. I profoundly love and accept myself, even with this resistance. I profoundly love and accept every single part of myself even with all of this resistance to change. And although I am now ready to let it go, I know that even if I don't let it go that I still completely love and accept every part of myself."

Move on to tapping point 9, the collarbone. You can tap on either side with all four fingers. Switch sides when you go through the tapping sequence the second time. Say out loud as you tap:

"But I am ready to let go of this remaining resistance and fear. I do not need it anymore. I can feel it leaving my body and I can feel the calm and peace coming into my body. I know this feeling of peacefulness. I know this feeling of calm. And I embrace these feelings within me now."

Move on to tapping point 10, under your arm. Tap on either side with all four fingers. Switch sides when you go through the tapping sequence the second time. Say out loud as you tap:

"I may still feel some resistance. I recognize it and I may feel it. But I will not criticize myself for having this resistance. I am choosing to just recognize that it is there and recognize how it feels. And it is OK. I love and accept myself even with this resistance and fear of change. I love and accept that it is my body trying to protect me. And I love and accept myself enough to let it go."

As always, assess your body and your feeling of resistance and reluctance to change on a scale of 1 to 10. If necessary, repeat the above tapping sequence a few times and at regular intervals until you have overcome your resistance.

Inaccurate targeting

Another of what I believe are the three most common problems that cause people to experience substandard results from their tapping is caused by inaccurately targeting your tapping. If this is the problem for you, it may be because your tapping script is too general. For example, suppose you are stressed and so you tap on stress using a tapping script that targets stress in general. This may work for you if you are experiencing a generally stressed out disposition. Even if the source of your stress is something more specific, you may still notice some positive results with a general script. Perhaps your stress would be at an eight out of ten level when you begin tapping and by tapping with a general tapping script you would be able to reduce it to a six out of ten.

If the type of stress you are experiencing is related to a specific concern, problem, or issue in your life however, you can likely achieve faster, better, more efficient results by drilling down on the specific issue that is causing the stress and then tapping on that specific issue.

If this is the type of problem that is getting in the way of successful tapping for you then the approach mentioned above about tapping on resistance is unlikely to work for you. That is because your problem is not resistance. It is not the case that your body is resisting letting go of a particular blockage. Your body may be quite ready to let go of the blockage. The problem is that your are not tapping on the blockage!

The solution to this problem, the way you can solve it is by thinking specifically about the issue that you want to tap on. Ask yourself questions like "what specifically is the problem?" "how did this specific problem arise in my life?" "what is my earliest memory of experiencing this specific problem?". Reviewing the chapter of this book on targeting your tapping will also be helpful for you in order to overcome this problem.

Previous memories

If you are not experiencing resistance to clearing a blockage, and your tapping script is well crafted and accurately targets the issue you wish to tap on, but you are *still* not experiencing the results you had hoped to achieve through tapping, the problem is most likely that you have some previous memory that is getting in the way. Basically what this means is that there is not just one source of the blockage, but there is actually two or more separate sources that are causing the same blockage. Suppose for example that you have a fear of public speaking and you wish to tap on this fear and overcome it. In an effort to drill down on the specific blockage you think back to an early memory of public speaking. Perhaps you gave answered a question out loud in front of the class when you were a child and you got the answer wrong and the class laughed at you. This is the sort of memory that might manifest into an emotional blockage that causes an intense fear of public speaking later in life. In many cases tapping on this issue and memory will help to clear the blockage and restore your body's natural energy flow. However, if there is a second memory that also accounts for your fear of public speaking then clearing the first memory but not the second is unlikely to fully resolve the blockage.

Suppose, for example, that in addition to the first memory described above, you also had an experience as a child where you swore or said an inappropriate word that was overheard by a teacher, a parent, or some adult in authority who punished you for this by washing your mouth out with soap and water. This might have been a very traumatic and embarrassing situation that could also manifest as an energy blockage causing a fear of public speaking in later life. In this situation there would actually be two traumatic memories, not just one, that are causing a single blockage. If you tap only on the memory of answering the question in class, or if you tap only on the memory of having your mouth washed out with soap, you are leaving the other memory untouched and thus still able to disrupt your equilibrium, preventing a full resolution of your fear of public speaking.

If this is your problem, you need to think carefully about your past, especially as a child, and recall other events that could be contributing to your blockages. Refer to the chapters in this book on targeting your tapping and developing your own tapping scripts in order to craft a tapping script that will deal with the secondary memory, then tap through that just as you did with the initial memory. In my experience, you will typically find that the two (or more) memories are not all of equal intensity. One is likely to be more responsible for the blockage than another. If you are experiencing problems in achieving the results in your tapping, and you have tried tapping on resistance as well as ensuring your tapping script is tight and accurate, tapping on secondary or tertiary memories is likely to improve your tapping results.

Tapping for children and teens

Studies have shown that teenagers experience a level of stress that is similar to adults. Children also suffer from stress, and although the evidence suggests it is at a lower rate than adults and teens, my own guess is that the stress children experience may be the most serious of all. This is because what happens to us in our early years can stick with us and alter our subconscious for the rest of our lives. Much of our character and personality is shaped in these first few years of life, as well as many of our most intractable energy blockages. EFT tapping is an excellent tool for breaking through these barriers as adults, but wouldn't it be even better if we could help our children to *never develop these blockages in the first place*?

The first question to ask in considering whether we can use EFT tapping with children in order to prevent them from experience subconscious physiological problems in their adult life. The answer is a resounding yes! EFT tapping can be just as effective for children as for adults. Indeed, EFT tapping can also be useful for pregnant women and their unborn children. While still in the womb, children are intimately connected and affected in some way by virtually everything that is felt and experienced by the mother. If the mother is suffering from emotional or physical distress, some of this will be passed on to the fetus. A pregnant mother who takes the time to tap through her problems and restore her internal equilibrium will pass this on to the unborn child as well.

Once the child is born and becomes verbal, they are in a position where they can learn to tap themselves. Although one of the great strengths of EFT tapping is that it is simple and accessible, I think that it is always helpful for everyone, especially children, to begin their exploration of EFT tapping with a facilitator. This could be a professional EFT practitioner, or it could be an interested parent who is comfortable with the idea and use of EFT tapping.

When it comes to introducing tapping to our children, there are basically two different types of approaches we could use. One is to tap for specific situations. For example if a child is having a temper tantrum, had a bad dream, or is late to achieve certain milestones such as bed-wetting. Another option is to use the general approach by tapping at regular intervals, regardless of any specific issues the child may or may not be experiencing at the time. This latter approach is useful for instilling the habit of tapping while a child is still young and increases the likelihood of them hanging on to this valuable tool for life. The former approach has more immediate utility in that it aims at dealing with situations that are (or will some become) out of control. Ultimately, I advocate using a mix of both approaches. For example a great way to introduce tapping can be as part of a ritual either when waking up or when going to bed. Consider the routine your child has before going to bed for example, such as using the bathroom, brushing his or her teeth, changing into pajamas, etc. Adding tapping into this routine can be a fun and effective way to encourage children to begin learning about and experimenting with tapping on their own.

One way a parent can facilitate this type of tapping is by having the child tell a story or share an emotion they experienced during their day. The child can share both positive and negative experiences as the parent can go through the tapping points on the child and have the child follow along. As the child gets older, the application of tapping scripts can be introduced and the child can learn to formulate his emotions and stories into a proper tapping script. Doing this routine before bed can be an effective strategy for preventing the long term damage that even minor emotional trauma can cause when experienced as a child. Just as brushing their teeth cleans away damaging residue from food and drink, tapping before bed cleans away potentially damaging residual emotions from the day and prepares them for a sound and healthy sleep.

Although it is unfortunately still very rare, I know there are some teachers that are working to integrate EFT tapping into part of childrens' school day. Some teachers introduce tapping at the beginning of the school year and then facilitate group tapping sessions shortly before an important test, public performance, or sometimes just as a quick tapping session after recess to refocus the student's minds and attention on their next tasks.

True tapping miracles: The young gangster

Throughout this book I've included a few stories that were told to me by friends, acquaintances, or clients that I have met. I've heard many remarkable stories over the years of the efficacy of EFT tapping and I've selected a small handful to present to you as part of this book. I have personally found these stories to be particularly uplifting and I share them with you in the hopes that they will inspire you on your wellness journey using EFT tapping.

A colleague of mine involved in researching energy psychology introduced me to a young man who shared a remarkable story about how his life changed when he discovered EFT tapping. His amazing story appears below, however please note that to protect his anonymity I have changed his name and some minor identifying details:

At only 16 years old, Deandre had already lived a hard life. He was born in poverty to a single mother in a neighborhood known for its high crime rate. He had four siblings who, together with himself and his mother, shared a small two bedroom apartment in a high rise housing project. Graffiti covered the interior corridors of the building. At night, gun shots could regularly be heard not too far in the distance. Deandre grew up in this world, knowing little else besides the streets. He started hanging around with some local gang members when he was only 13 years old. By 16 he had dropped out of high school and was selling crack cocaine on the street in a what was essentially an open-air drug market in an impoverished part of a major American city.

"It was crazy man, just crazy," Deandre recalls of his time running with his gang. "Like, when you're that age man, you just think you're invincible. You think nothing can touch you. You got a strap, you got your boys, and it's like, come at me! What are you going to do? I'm the king of this corner!"

But within only a few years of working as a street-level drug dealer Deandre had seen close friends, teenagers like him, lose their lives to bullets from a gun, long prison sentences for drug trafficking and gun crimes, and to the horrors of drug addiction. It didn't take an expert or a social worker to tell that Deandre was on the road to a very troubled future, if he had any future at all. Deandre began to see it too.

"There was this one guy, kind of new to the streets you know. He came back a bit light on a package you know, like maybe $50 short or something. It was the second time he was short and some of the boys took him back behind some old buildings and just lit him up. He never walked again after that. And these were his own boys! They shot him, crippled him for life, over $50! That's when I knew that the life I was living and the choices I was making had to change. That s--- was crazy man. I had to get out of that."

The problem for Deandre was that leaving the gang was easier said than done. It was the only life Deandre knew. He had no education, no skills, no legitimate work history, and no money. He knew he was headed for a dead end but the inertia driving him felt like too much for him to overcome. He didn't know how he could turn things around.

One afternoon Deandre was on his corner, selling drugs as he did most days. The sky opened up and it started to pour. Thunder crashed overhead as Deandre ran down the street and ducked into a local Chinese restaurant to grab some food and wait for the rain to pass. Little did Deandre know, this afternoon would be a turning point in his life. As he say eating his food a small TV was on in the corner playing some daytime talk show. As fate would have it, the guest on the talk show that day was talking about EFT tapping and how it could be used for therapeutic purposes and to make major changes in one's life.

"I wasn't paying any mind to it at first," Deandre smiles, "but then this dude started banging his fingers on his face and his chest and I was like, what the hell is this?!" Deandre watched as the guest showed the host of the show and the audience how to tap. The guest went on to explain the amazing changes that tapping could facilitate and how simple it was to start tapping on one's problems.

"I was like, I ain't never seen nothing like that but if it works for them, maybe it could work for me too. I was desperate at that time and I was ready to do whatever if I thought it could get me out from where I was," Deandre explains. He got up from the table and went to the small, dirty washroom of the restaurant. There in that washroom, the dim incandescent bulb reflecting off the grimy tiled wall, Deandre tapped through his first EFT tapping session, whispering the tapping script to himself as best as he could remember it.

"I felt better," Deandre describes. "It's not like all my problems were just behind me or nothing. But like, there was a focus to my mind you know? Like I could think about problems as if I was above them looking down. Not like they were just buzzing all around me and taking over my mind."

Deandre tapped daily from that day forward. He would tap secretly, usually in washrooms or whenever he was alone and no one was watching. He felt embarrassed to be doing something that looked so silly but he knew he had to continue with tapping because he could feel it working. He could feel his inner strength growing with each tapping session. He also felt himself gaining a mental clarity and perspective that he had previously lacked. For the first time in his life, Deandre felt that there might be a way out of poverty and gang life.

Secretly, Deandre began saving small amounts of money he earned from dealing. He hid the bills in a sock in his dresser drawer in the room he shared with two of siblings. He wasn't exactly sure what he was going to do with it except that it would be for getting him out of the projects, out of the gang, and on the road to a better life.

About three months after discovering tapping, with a few hundred dollars secretly stuffed in a sock at home, Deandre's opportunity came. He got a call from an old friend who grew up in the same building as Deandre. Deandre's friend had avoided gang life when his family moved to the west coast a few years ago. Deandre's friend was a couple of years older than him. He had just finished high school and had been accepted at a local state college. Deandre confided in his friend that he wanted to make a big change in his life and was worried where he would end up if he didn't do it soon. Deandre's friend understood his situation and offered to let him stay with him for a few months out west. Deandre seized the opportunity. He bought a bus ticket the following day, said goodbye to his family, and left his old life miles behind him.

When he arrived in California, Deandre kept tapping his way through his problems and his mental and emotional blockages. He landed an entry level job at a local restaurant and although it didn't pay much it was enough for him to rent a room in a clean and safe house within a month. Deandre worked long hours and didn't have much, but for once he had safety and security. He had a future that didn't involve prison, addiction or death. To Deandre, that was much more than he had only a few months prior.

Today, not even two years later, Deandre still works at that same restaurant except now he is an assistant manager. He has a girlfriend, good friends, and recently completed his high school equivalency. Deandre plans to apply to college next year.

"For me, tapping was the ladder that I climbed to get out of all that craziness I was caught up with before. I don't know where I'd be without tapping. Maybe dead. Maybe in jail. I don't know and I don't want to know. I'm excited for the future now," Deandre says beaming, "you come talk to me in another year and see where I'm at."

PART III: Transform your life with EFT tapping

Mindset shifting for increased self-esteem

Many times when people look at their lives, they are able to readily identify problems or emotional issues that they are suffering from. I have found that sometimes when people start moving forward on making changes they quit before they achieve complete success. Sometimes this is because they become scared, or because they feel as though they are losing something.

The things in our lives that are from the past, even things we don't like, often become a part of our identity. Our past events shape us in a truly fundamental way that can endure over time and indeed throughout one's entire life. Trying to purge aspects of one's core identity can be overwhelming and intimidating and may make us want to seek comfort in the familiar rather than pressing forward through positive changes in our lives.

A point that must be raised for consideration here however, is that just because events endure in our memories and our identities through time, it does not mean that the *meaning* of these events must forever remain fixed. The way that we think of our past events and the implications of these events to our character and ourselves as human beings is not something that is forever set in stone. Meaning, understanding, and representation can all be shifting, transient concepts when we are willing to apply the necessary mental work to shift our mindset out of the old and into the new. The way you represent a past pain or hurt for example can be shifted over time such that you come to identify that aspect of your past not as a time of being a victim, or as an indication that you have a weak character or are easily taken advantage of. Rather, your perception of this part of yourself could be shifted to one of strength. A painful past event can be representative of your ability to overcome adversity; to survive and to thrive in the face of challenges.

When you start to change you internal representations in this way, you shift all available information in your conscious memory towards the new and more positive change you wish to make. Every image, sound, smell, detail, feeling etc that is playing out in your memory in relation to this event must be scrutinized and shifted piece by piece into the new broader puzzle of understanding the memory in a positive way and from a position of strength. Everything inside your memory is a *present and current* part of how you perceive your identity. While the events may be in the past and unable to be changed, your perceptions and understanding is playing out right now, in the present. That is what you can change.

When I explain this concept to people they sometimes ask "who will I be after I change these memories?" This is certainly a legitimate question and speaks to the degree of fear so many of us harbor over potential changes in our lives. People worry whether they will be an entirely different person following such mindset shifts directed at key events in their lives that have come to shape their identities.

For people with such concerns, I have good news. You will still very much be yourself. You will always be you. But you will be a happier you. A more content and at peace you. You will be you, but with increased self-esteem and a healthier, more positive outlook on life. When you change your understanding of past painful events, you will self-actualize who you are and what you want for yourself. You will in some sense, be more "you" than ever before!

Losing weight with EFT tapping

Today's modern world is one where calories are essentially free. Processed fast food is sold on virtually every street corner in major urban centers. We are marketed to relentlessly by huge corporate conglomerates whose sole job in life is to induce you to come in to their restaurant or take a swing by their drive through window and eat another cheeseburger, or piece of fried chicken, or whatever special they are selling this month. The food often tastes pretty good and is sold pretty cheaply. In the short-term, it seems like not such a bad deal to grab that fast food combo for dinner. And then why not upsize it for an extra 40 cents?

Add to this, the fact that people are working longer hours than they were a generation ago. The rise of convenient technology like the internet, email, and smart phones, means that we are always reachable and always available to work on something. Even when it is not work, our time is increasingly filled by these new technologies in a way that doesn't leave us with seemingly any free time to ourselves. The result of this is a massive spike in the level of stress the current Western population deals with in a typical day. This increase in stress is a huge problem in itself, to be sure. But another subsequent problem caused by stress is a lack of will power and a lack of time to prepare and eat healthy meals with our families.

These two factors, the incredible availability of cheap, easy, and convenient calories combined with rising stress levels that are common in our modern lives creates the perfect storm the obesity epidemic we are currently seeing sweep the Western developed world. The United States has led the pack with our ever expanding waist lines, but we are certainly not alone in our losing battle of the bulge. Obesity is a serious and all too common problem affecting millions and millions across the globe. We need a solution, and we need it soon.

Is EFT tapping the solution that can permanently solve humanities collective weight problem? I am optimistic that it can be. To be clear, there are many different aspects that must all come together for successful weight loss and permanent weight maintenance and control. Despite what anyone may tell you, there really is no single magic bullet that will make permanent weight management a reality. No fancy juice, milk shake, exercise machine, or bizarre fad diet will by itself be a permanent weight loss solution. A multifaceted approach is necessary for most people. Where EFT tapping comes in is as a fundamental, core part of healthy living. You might think of a commitment to EFT tapping as the trunk of the tree that supports the various branches, all of which contribute to losing weight.

One of the great things about EFT tapping is how quickly it can work to solve many of the problems in your life. But let's be clear, you didn't develop you weight problem in one week and you will not solve it in one week either. EFT tapping can be a core part of your permanent weight solution, as it has for hundreds of others, many of whom I have personally met through coaching and seminars. But success, especially lasting and permanent success, entails a commitment on your part to regularly tap through the issues that have contributed to your weight gain.

To begin your weight loss journey with EFT tapping, you'll want to think about some of your past experiences and beliefs about food. We all have subconscious programming about food. It is important to point out however that this is not always negative. If you have met someone who seems to effortlessly maintain a healthy weight, it is likely that they have subconscious programming about food that is positive and works in their favor. They are probably totally unaware of the programming that is operating behind their subconscious mind because they have never thought about it. It has never been a problem for them and so they've never focused any attention on it. If you have a weight problem however, it is important that you do focus on you subconscious programming and come to understand what values, beliefs, and emotions you have about food and what is being triggered in your mind when you eat the foods you eat.

You also need to pay attention to your subconscious programming about weight loss itself. I have found that for many people who are overweight or obese, their subconscious programming is telling them that losing weight is very difficult, maybe impossible. Their programming tells them they will do it, one day, but it will be surely be very hard and unpleasant.

All the years we have had this negative subconscious programming are years that we have been bombarded with self-destructive values about eating, being healthy, and losing weight. Our subconscious programming can create an inertia over time that drives us towards the wrong choices. It keeps us going back to the buffet line even when we're already full. It keeps us filling up the cart at the grocery store with chips, soda, and snacks that we know aren't good for us at all. It causes us to think of healthy food as bland, lacking flavor, being totally undesirable except for it's nutrients. And it reinforces the fact that that weight loss is just too hard for us to take on today. Maybe some other day we will, but not today.

As part of your efforts to understand and re-tune your subconscious programming, consider the messages you are receiving from the media about food and weight loss. Too often, the problem of weight loss is made out to be a math problem. Take in fewer calories than you burn and you will lose weight. Eat more carbs and less fat. Or eat more fat and less carbs. Eat "paleo" food like a caveman. Eat raw food like a herbivore. The messages are mixed, confusing, and rarely helpful.

The fact is that losing weight and maintaining a healthy weight is about more than just what you eat or how you exercise. You need to develop new and healthy habits while tapping through your emotional blockages about your weight and your damaging relationship with food. Find habits that work for you. If you are not a "gym person" then don't buy a gym membership! Find other ways you can exercise instead, like walking the dog, riding a bike, or playing with your kids. Whatever sounds enjoyable to you is much more likely to be something you can successfully incorporate as a "branch" in your "tree" of health and weight loss.

As you start to think about some of these things that are holding you back from your weight loss goals and how you can start thinking about exercise and healthy living as an enjoyable, on-going journey, rather than a difficult and fearsome struggle, you should begin tapping out some of these old blockages to get your body's energy flowing freely through your body, inspiring further change and progress towards healthy living. Here is a tapping script you can use as you begin this journey.

Before we begin the tapping sequence find somewhere comfortable to sit. You can sit in a chair, or on the floor, whichever is more comfortable for you. If you choose to sit in the floor it may be helpful to sit on a cushion or some padding. You can lean up against a wall or sit in the middle of the room. Sit cross-legged if you like. All that matters about how you sit is that you keep your back straight. Do not slouch while going through the tapping sequence. Remove your glasses if you wear them, and any jewelry that could interfere with the tapping sequence.

Rate how you feel about your efforts to lose weight. Use a scale of 1 to 10 with 1 being perfectly comfortable and happy with your weight loss efforts and 10 being maximum dissatisfaction with your weight loss efforts. It is important to take this initial benchmark of the level of comfort you feel about your weight loss efforts. After the tapping sequence is complete, you will ask yourself this same question again. Typically when tapping for weight loss I find clients experience at least a 1 or 2 point decrease with each tapping sequence. Often the decrease is more significant than that, such as 3 or 4 points. Sometimes even just a single tapping sequence can reduce discomfort by more than 4 points. If you don't notice a change after the initial tapping sequence, you can try going through the entire sequence again from the beginning, or refer to the chapter in this book on what to do if tapping isn't working for you.

Remember that the more in tune you are with your body before you begin the tapping sequence the more effective tapping can be. Take a moment to review the chapter about what to do before you begin tapping. Take ownership over your emotional well being. *You* are in control. It is *your* energy and it belongs only to you. No one else can control your energy. Only you can.

If you would benefit from a visual aid as you proceed through this tapping sequence, remember that I have prepared a free video demonstration for readers of this book. If you think this would be helpful for you, please visit my website at **www.randallawrence.com** to get access to this free video and use it to help you tap through this sequence.

Start by tapping with four fingers on point 1, the side of your hand (or the "karate chop" point). Tap gently. There is no need to be hostile with yourself or hurt yourself. Say out loud:

"Even though I am feeling disappointed about my efforts to lose weight in the past, I profoundly and completely love and accept myself. I profoundly love and accept the way I feel right now. I profoundly love and accept myself and everything that I am."

Move on to tapping on point 2, your inner wrist. You can tap with two fingers, four fingers, or your opposite wrist. Say out loud:

"Even though I feel shame and disappointment about my weight. Even though sometimes I think I will always be overweight. Even though sometimes I feel like I can't lose weight because it is too hard for me. Even though I feel this way, I profoundly love and accept myself, and my body, and the way it feels right now."

Move on to tapping point 3, the top of your head. Tap with all four fingers on both hands and say out loud:

"I love the way my body feels right now. I know my body responds this way to try to protect me. I know that my feelings of disappointment about my weight and my weight loss efforts are my body's way of making sure I pay attention to my health. I love and accept that my body wants me to be safe from harm. I am profoundly grateful for this reaction. I love and accept every part of my body and I love and accept all of the things it does for me."

Move on to tapping point 4, your eyebrows. You can tap on either side with two fingers. Switch sides when you go through the tapping sequence the second time. Say out loud as you tap:

"I know what it feels like to overcome my challenges. To do things I thought I was not capable of. I know what it feels like to be achieve a goal I set for myself. I love and accept that my body wants me to achieve my weight loss goal. Even though I have this shame and disappointment in myself for my past failures in maintaining a healthy weight, I know what my success will look like and feel like."

Move on to tapping point 5, the side of your eye. Tap with two fingers on either side. When you go through the tapping sequence the second time you can switch sides. Say out loud as you tap:

"I am open to achieving my weight loss goal as I move through my blockages and disturbances, releasing myself from this shame and disappointment. I know I can do it. I know I can restore my body's naturally peaceful flow of energy."

Move on to tapping point 6, under your eye. Tap with two fingers on either side. When you go through the tapping sequence the second time you can switch sides. Say out loud as you tap:

"I have control over my body. I have control over my emotions. I have control over all of my feelings. I have control over the way my energy flows. I am in control and no one else can control me. I can feel my strength to achieve my weight loss goal rising within me. I can feel my energy starting to flow as the blockages and disturbances become smaller and smaller."

Move on to tapping point 7, under your nose. Tap with two fingers and say out loud as you tap:

"This remaining shame and disappointment about being overweight is hard to let go of. I understand that my body does not want me to let it go. I understand that my body wants to keep me safe. I know and appreciate all my body does for me. And I've spent so much time believing that I couldn't do it. That I couldn't achieve my weight loss goals and live a healthy life."

Move on to tapping point 8, your chin. Tap with two fingers and say out loud as you tap:

"But now I love and accept that my body responds this way. I profoundly love and accept myself, even with this shame and disappointment in myself for being overweight. I profoundly love and accept every single part of myself and I know that I am strong enough to lose weight. I know that the love and acceptance I have for myself and my body will give me the strength that I need to lose weight."

Move on to tapping point 9, your collarbone. You can tap on either side with all four fingers. Switch sides when you go through the tapping sequence the second time. Say out loud as you tap:

"I am ready to let go of this remaining disappointment about my inability to lose weight. I do not need that disappointment anymore. I am strong and I will succeed at losing weight. I can feel the disappointment and shame leaving my body. I can feel my strength and commitment to lose weight increasing within me. I know this feeling of strength. I know what it feels like to achieve my goals. I know what it feels like to overcome my challenges and I embrace these feelings within me now."

Move on to tapping point 10, under your arm. Tap on either side with all four fingers. Switch sides when you go through the tapping sequence the second time. Say out loud as you tap:

"I may still some shame and disappointment in my previous efforts to lose weight. I recognize that and I may feel it. But I will not criticize myself for having these feelings. I am choosing to just recognize that they are there and recognize how they feel. And it is OK. I love and accept myself. I love and accept that it is my body trying to protect me. And I love and accept myself enough to lose weight."

Take a deep breath in and let it out. Then ask yourself again, on a scale of 1 to 10 how you feel about your efforts to lose weight? Do you feel stronger now? Do you feel empowered to lose weight? Go through the tapping sequence again from the beginning if you're still not sure that you have the personal strength to achieve your weight loss goals.

True tapping miracles: the yo-yo dieter

Throughout this book I've included a few stories that were told to me by friends, acquaintances, or clients that I have met. I've heard many remarkable stories over the years of the efficacy of EFT tapping and I've selected a small handful to present to you as part of this book. I have personally found these stories to be particularly uplifting and I share them with you in the hopes that they will inspire you on your wellness journey using EFT tapping.

Marcy was a client of mine who had struggled with her weight and body issue for years. I asked her for permission to share her story with you and she agreed. Her is Marcy's story of success using EFT tapping:

Marcy was a dieting expert. She could tell you exactly how what you were and were not allowed to eat on the South Beach Diet. She had an encyclopedic understanding of the Four Hour Body's diet and exercise commandments. She had mastered the Paleo and Keto diets. For a time she ate nothing but bananas and multivitamins. At one time or another Marcy had tried virtually every diet under the sun. Some of them worked for her and some of them didn't. Some of them made her feel great, others made her feel sick and unhealthy. But whatever the diet, they all had one thing in common: within a few months of trying it, she was right back to where she was before.

Marcy's weight was like a yo-yo. Whenever it dropped, it would always spring right back up again. Marcy had no problem trying diets. She had no problem experiencing success with some diets either. Her problem was maintaining her weight loss beyond just a few months at a time.

When I met Marcy she was completely demoralized. She felt that she had tried everything and that nothing would work for her in the lasting way that she wanted. And indeed she had in fact tried just about every diet out there. I've never met someone who could say they committed so much time and energy to dieting as Marcy. And yet sitting there in my office, she presented as a clearly overweight and emotionally distraught woman. A master dieter who for all her efforts was still overweight.

I knew Marcy's problem had to be in her subconscious programming. Her willpower and her conscious, focused effort on dieting suggested to me that the solution for her was going to be resolving some deep emotional blockages. The solution certainly wasn't just trying another diet, she had already been doing that for years and achieved only short-term success at best, and headaches, stomach pains, and emotional turmoil at worst.

We began by discussing Marcy's previous experiences and values surrounding food. I was trying to find something that might have happened in her life, likely in childhood, that would account for the disruption in her emotional energy and her unhealthy subconscious programming about food. After some discussion, she recalled how her mother would always insist that the family ate all of the food they were served for a meal. Her mother would claim that because children in poor countries were starving, no one in their family should waste food. "Good children clean their plates" she would tell Marcy and her siblings dogmatically.

This is a common and seemingly innocent enough edict, however for Marcy it planted a kernel of what would come to be an unhealthy value system relating to food and eating that would play out in her subconscious every time she ate something. Dieting and restricting caloric intake would sometimes necessarily involve not eating everything she was served, such as at a restaurant, a friend's house, or a social function. Although she couldn't put her finger on the cause, this would trigger feelings of guilt and tension within her. On the one hand, she wanted to stick to her diet. On the other hand, she didn't want to waste food. She identified as a good person and since she had internalized her mother's values about wasting food she was frequently confronted with irreconcilable choices between following her diet and not wasting food.

It was this internal tension that would drive Marcy away from every diet she had tried within a few weeks or months. People had told her it must just be a lack of will power, but I knew this couldn't be it. She always had the will power to study new diets, start new ones, cycle through old ones. Marcy had no issues with will power. Marcy had an issue with negative subconscious programming.

We tapped together on this deep emotional blockage Marcy was experiencing and right away she told me she felt a change within her that she couldn't fully describe. She said she felt more clear-headed and in control of things. We tapped together regularly for a few months, and Marcy reported she was having no problem at all sticking to a regular diet routine that was healthy and enjoyable for her. Within six months, Marcy had lost over 50 pounds and was back to a healthy weight again. I encouraged her to continue with her tapping routine to prevent falling back into the same problems she had experienced previously.

About 18 months later I saw Marcy again and she looked great! She had maintained her healthy weight and felt great about herself. She told me that she didn't even feel like she was on a diet at all. She had developed the strength and discipline to eat healthy foods most of the time, exercise when she felt like it, and even ate the odd bit of junk food sometimes when she really wanted a treat. What she had needed during all those years of yo-yo dieting wasn't a better diet or an extra shot of will power, it was an internal clearing of the emotional and mental blockages that were holding her back. EFT tapping was the tool that she needed to lose weight and maintain it effortlessly.

Controlling cravings and addictions

What is addiction?

We human beings are remarkably susceptible to addiction. Collectively, we always have been and probably always will be. There is something about us, the way we are wired, our body chemistry, the things we like and dislike, and the habits we develop through life that make us all as human beings easy targets for certain temptations that exist in the world. These temptations are not the same for all of us. Some people are alcoholics while others can drink occasionally without problems. Some people are addicted to smoking while others have found the strength to quit forever. Some people suffer from addictions that play out within a certain social context, such as an addiction to rage. Others are addicted to work.

Addictions come in all shapes and sizes but what they have in common is their negative, overpowering influence on our lives. Many of us know personally what it means to be in the grip of an addiction, either because we have suffered through one ourselves, either in the past or the present, or perhaps because we have watched a friend, family member, or loved one battle with the demons of addiction.

Whether it is an addiction to sugary foods, or crack-cocaine, the thoughts, feelings, and actions that addictions cause in our bodies and brains are all very similar.

My interest in using EFT tapping as a cure for addictions comes from my background and research into using EFT tapping to conquer cravings for junk food. During my process of researching the topic of weight loss I would often encounter people who had the attitude that weight loss was easy. "Just stop eating!" they would say, as if these words would be a magic bullet to anyone struggling with their weight. I have heard the same thing said about alcoholics. "Just stop drinking!"

The fact is however, that such a directive alone is absolutely useless and anyone who has dealt with a weight problem or an alcohol addiction knows that. The reason they are useless is because there is so much more going on "behind the scenes" that accounts for our out of control cravings. The well-intentioned folks who yell at the addict to simply stop their damaging behavior may as well be yelling at a ball rolling down a hill or a rock falling of a cliff. They can yell "stop" as loud and as often as they want, but it won't stop anything at all.

As I started digging into these topics, the common root of all addictions became increasingly obvious. Smoking, drinking, eating, drugs, procrastination, you name it. These addictions are all essentially "escapism". It is our attempt, often subconsciously, to avoid dealing with a particular reality that we are unaccustomed to, dislike, or are scared of. We will do anything to avoid whatever it is that is bothering us, and that drives us deeper in to the depths of addiction.

If a feeling, or a thought, pops into your head while you are trying to focus on something else, do you let it divert your attention? Sometimes, maybe, but mostly you don't. You put the distraction aside, or in the back of your thoughts, and focus on what you were doing. We all have some basic mechanism for doing this that we have developed over time. But the basic mechanism that we develop without really trying is not a perfect one. That is why we sometimes get so distracted that we lose focus entirely on what we were doing. The mechanism has its limits and those limits define where your own internal power ends and gives way to some other external power. That external power can take the form of a person saying something to you that stir emotions that distract you from your thoughts. It could take the form of bad news, good news, a particular smell or sight that is of significance, or something else entirely. But whatever it is, and to whatever extent you are unable to deal with it, you are essentially rendered powerless in the face of something greater than yourself. When you lose the power or control over yourself that you are naturally endowed with, and when that loss of control causes a negative impact in your life, you may be experiencing an addiction.

In our minds, we have programs running all the time, like software on a computer. We could think of them as pictures, or movies, or slide shows. There are always memories moving around in our mind, either in the forefront or somewhere in the back. This is most noticeable when we are trying to sleep and for the most part, we have no real concept of what causes this or how to control it. You probably don't know how to change the memories or "movies" that are playing out in your own mind at any given time, just as most people don't know how to gain control over their addictions.

At the end of the day, we are all the same in that we are all powerless over something. The limits of our own power and agency over ourselves is what sets us apart. In this respect, our self-control, our willpower, our self-discipline, and ultimately our ability to overcome the addictions that drag us down is like a muscle. If left untrained it will be small and weak. Our domain of power and control over ourselves will be small too. But as we put in the hard but worthwhile work of strengthening that muscle, our control grows and grows, until we can stare down the things that held us powerless before and know that they are nothing to us now. That we can conquer them because we have become great and stronger than their negative power over us. This is what it means to conquer addiction.

Disconnecting painful past memories from present day actions

If I had the same experiences and the same thoughts throughout my life as you have in yours, I have no doubt that today I would act just like you. I am just as sure that the reverse is true as well. Our current actions, both positive and negative, are based on our previous experiences, feelings, and memories, and the effect these things have had on us.

Sometimes when I talk about previous experiences and memories with a client during a coaching session they get uncomfortable. Lots of us don't like dealing with the pain in our past any more than we like dealing with the pain in our future. But it is crucial to dig deeply into these past events to clear our blockages and the things that are holding us back. Sometimes we need to take a step back before we can run forward.

Being ready to conquer your addictions means being ready to face head on the things that have hurt you in the past. You need to face them first of all, and then second of all you need to work to change them. This is hard. It is much easier to just keep doing what we're doing. It is easier to keep smoking, drinking, yelling, eating, or whatever other destructive behavior our habits dictate that we must participate in. Many of us would much rather stick to the familiar than to brave the hurt and pain of our past. We are conditioned to act and behave in these ways without ever thinking about it. When you hear a certain thing, or you're in a certain situation, that triggers something for you, such as the sight of an alcohol commercial or the smell of a cigarette, we are triggered like Pavlov's dog into losing control over ourselves and our minds and fixating on what we expect to come next.

Inside of us we have memories recorded throughout our lives. These memories to a large extent control our thoughts, feelings, and actions in the present day. Let me share with you an example of what I am talking about. When I was about 10 years old, I recall being involved in a school yard fight. A number of other kids ganged up on me and tried to beat me up. I was scared and ran from them but they caught up to me and beat me with a branch from a tree. It was painful and frightening for me at that age and for a long time after. But when I tell you this story today, it no longer affects me emotionally. It did for a long time, but it does not now. It doesn't, because if I let it, who is the person beating me with a stick today? It isn't the 10 year old boys on the school yard. It is me. I am only beating up myself when I dwell on this memory and allow it to dictate any of my thoughts, actions, or feelings in the present day.

When I made the analogy earlier about "movies" playing out in our brain, this is what I mean. There is a movie of myself getting beaten on the school yard. But it is only a movie. And not only is it a movie, but I am the movie director. I am the one who controls it and not the other way around. Further, as much as they may control us, memories are not real things. They are only memories. The real events already occurred in the past, maybe the very distant past. There is no necessity in letting our painful memories control us. We can decouple them from thinking and acting in the present and leave them there. They may always exist in our heads but they do not always need to dictate our actions.

I have worked to overcome my own addictions, and decouple my painful past memories from the driving force behind actions in my present day life. And there is no difference between me and you. I am not smarter, better, or special in any way. The only difference is that I have discovered the techniques needed to conquer cravings and addictions once and for all. Once you discover and master the same technique, you too will have this same inner strength.

What is the connection between memories and addictions?

I want to make sure I take the time necessary to explain why memories are important in the context of addiction. Too often, people do not appreciate the connection between the two. They certainly get little help from the typical medical establishment view of addictions as something boiled down to a chemical problem that can often be dealt with by (surprise!) prescription medication. In some cases this might be effective but my research and experience suggests than in the vast majority of cases there is a better way.

The reason memories are important is that they account for the blockages that exist within us, impeding the proper flow of energy through our bodies. When our energy cannot flow the way it is meant to, we lose our natural equilibrium. We become increasingly driven away from our goals and the things that make us happy and healthy in life. We may still achieve some of these things, but we can never reach our true potential. Just as a tree that is forced to grow very close to the brick wall of a building, its roots will be impacted and its growth will be stunted. It may still reach a considerable height and strength, but it will be smaller and weaker than it could have been without that wall next to it.

EFT tapping is the easiest, best, most effective method I have ever heard of for breaking through the "walls" that are inhibiting our growth and limiting our potential.

When we tap on our blockages in conjunction with a proper tapping script, we can chip away at that blockage, ultimately clearing it entirely and restoring the natural energy flow that our bodies are meant to have. Will power, self-esteem, and the ability to turn away from our bad habits all follow from our actualized self. We are not born with addictions. They develop over time as a product of our life experiences and the blockages they cause. EFT tapping is the tool that in a sense allows us to turn back the clock on addiction, to a time before the natural energy flowing through the body was impaired and to a time when we were not held as a prisoner in the cage of an addiction.

Applying EFT tapping to addiction recovery

By tapping on our damaging memories and present day addictions we can begin to change the way we perceive these memories as well as the effect they have on us today and in the future. We can't change the actual event that happened of course, that is in the past and it is set in stone. But that doesn't matter. What matters for our lives going forward is how we remember it.

As always, before you begin tapping take a moment to get in tune with your body. On a scale of 1 to 10 rate the discomfort your addiction is presently causing you. It may also be helpful to review the chapter about what to do before you begin tapping prior to starting this session. As you tap through your addiction, always remember that *you* are in control here. It is *your* energy and it belongs only to you.

If you would benefit from a visual aid as you proceed through this tapping sequence, remember that I have prepared a free video demonstration for readers of this book. If you think this would be helpful for you, please visit my website at **www.randallawrence.com** to get access to this free video and use it to help you tap through this sequence.

Start by tapping with four fingers on point 1, the side of your hand (or the "karate chop" point). Tap gently. There is no need to be hostile with yourself or hurt yourself. Say out loud:

"Even though I am feeling that my addiction is out of control right now, I profoundly and completely love and accept myself. I profoundly love and accept the way I feel right now. I profoundly love and accept myself and everything that I am."

Move on to tapping on point 2, your inner wrist. You can tap with two fingers, four fingers, or your opposite wrist. Say out loud:

"Even though I feel shame and disappointment over my addiction and my inability to control it. Even though sometimes I think I will always be addicted. Even though sometimes I feel like I can't conquer this addiction because I am too weak and it is too strong. Even though I feel this way right now, I profoundly love and accept myself, my body, and my mind, and the way I feel right now."

Move on to tapping point 3, the top of your head. Tap with all four fingers on both hands and say out loud:

"I love the way my body feels right now. I know my body only wants what is best for me. I know my mind only wants what is best for me. I know that my feelings of shame and disappointment about my addiction is my body's way of making sure I pay attention to my health and wellness. I love and accept that my body wants me to be safe from harm. I am profoundly grateful for this reaction. I love and accept every part of my body and I love and accept all of the things it does for me."

Move on to tapping point 4, your eyebrows. You can tap on either side with two fingers. Switch sides when you go through the tapping sequence the second time. Say out loud as you tap:

"I know what it feels like to overcome my challenges. To do things I thought I was not capable of. I know what it feels like to be achieve a goal I set for myself. I love and accept that my body wants me to conquer this addiction. Even though I have this shame and disappointment in myself for allowing my addiction to spiral out of control, I know what my success will look like and feel like."

Move on to tapping point 5, the side of your eye. Tap with two fingers on either side. When you go through the tapping sequence the second time you can switch sides. Say out loud as you tap:

"I want to be well and healthy again. Free of addiction just as I am intended to be. I can feel myself moving through my blockages and disturbances, releasing myself from this shame and disappointment of addiction. I know I can do it. I know I can restore my body's naturally peaceful flow of energy."

Move on to tapping point 6, under your eye. Tap with two fingers on either side. When you go through the tapping sequence the second time you can switch sides. Say out loud as you tap:

"I have control over my body. I have control over my emotions. I have control over all of my feelings. I have control over the way my energy flows. I am in control and no one else can control me. I can feel my strength rising within me. I know I am stronger than this addiction. I can feel beyond a shadow of a doubt that I can beat this. I can feel my energy starting to flow as the blockages and disturbances become smaller and smaller."

Move on to tapping point 7, under your nose. Tap with two fingers and say out loud as you tap:

"This remaining shame and disappointment about being addicted is hard to let go of. I understand that my body does not want me to let it go. I understand that my body wants to keep me safe. I know and appreciate all my body does for me. And I've spent so much time believing that I couldn't do it. That I couldn't beat this addiction and live a healthy life."

Move on to tapping point 8, your chin. Tap with two fingers and say out loud as you tap:

"But now I love and accept that my body responds this way. I profoundly love and accept myself, even with this addiction and all the shame and difficulty it has brought into my life. I profoundly love and accept every single part of myself and I know that I am strong enough to make my own choices. I know that the love and acceptance I have for myself will give me the strength that I need to conquer this addiction."

Move on to tapping point 9, your collarbone. You can tap on either side with all four fingers. Switch sides when you go through the tapping sequence the second time. Say out loud as you tap:

"I am ready to let go of this remaining compulsion to engage in destructive behavior. I do not need that negativity in my life anymore. I am strong and I will succeed in living an addiction free life. I can feel the disappointment and shame leaving my body. I can feel my strength and commitment to my health and well-being rising within me. I know this feeling of strength. I know what it feels like to achieve my goals. I know what it feels like to overcome my challenges and I embrace these feelings within me now."

Move on to tapping point 10, under your arm. Tap on either side with all four fingers. Switch sides when you go through the tapping sequence the second time. Say out loud as you tap:

"I may still some difficulty controlling cravings and giving into addiction. I recognize that and I may feel it. But I will not criticize myself for having these feelings. I am choosing to just recognize that they are there and recognize how they feel. And it is OK. I love and accept myself. I love and accept that it is my body trying to protect me. And I love and accept myself enough to live my life without addictions."

Take a deep breath in and let it out. Then ask yourself again, on a scale of 1 to 10 how you feel about your ability to control an addiction? Do you feel stronger now? Do you feel empowered to make the choices you want to make? Go through the tapping sequence again from the beginning if you're still not sure that you have the personal strength you will need. When you are feeling weak again, repeat the tapping sequence. That could be next week, it could be tomorrow, or it could be five minutes from now. Over time, the compulsion will fade and the addiction will weaken as your body's natural energy equilibrium is restored. Think of your tapping sessions as a pressure hose, chipping off old, dried up, peeling paint that is your addiction. The hose may not get all of the dried up old paint off the first time. But each time you chip away at more and more, you can feel the difference in your life as you move steadily towards the life you desire for yourself.

Remember also that the more specific you can be in your tapping about the memories you think may be contributing to your addiction the better. I encourage you to take some time and really think about why you are where you are and why you are doing the things you are doing. Modify the tapping sequence according to your own needs by referring to the chapters on targeting your tapping and developing your own tapping scripts in order to further enhance your tapping experience.

EFT Tapping to Cure Anxiety

Anxiety is, or at least can be, a normal response to stressful situations and experiencing anxiety is a normal part of being human. Anxiety can become a disorder however, when you experience anxiety repeatedly in situations where it is not productive or rational. Anxiety is remarkably common in our modern world. Studies indicate that 1 out of every 4 people will at some point in their lives experience a diagnosable anxiety disorder. Anxiety disorders are no doubt a part of your life, either because you have a friend or loved one who has, is, or will experience one, or because you personally struggle with an anxiety disorder.

The classic example of an anxiety inducing situation is public speaking. Most people experience some level of anxiety about the thought of giving a speech or a presentation in front of a large group of people. If the anxiety is unwelcome and gets in the way of the performing well, or inhibits the person from agreeing to give speeches or presentations in the future, it could rightly be classified as a disorder. It would be a disorder in this situation because the fear is irrational and overblown, and also because the anxiety comes to form a life obstacle. Many people sacrifice success in their careers, relationships, and other aspects of life, in favor of giving into their anxiety disorder.

Anxiety can manifest in numerous ways. It can take the form of thoughts, such as thinking about problems or consequences for actions that are detached from reality. For example someone who is experiencing anxiety related to giving a speech might have thoughts that are myopically focused on possible negative outcomes. They might think through all the different ways they could screw the speech up, how the audience would laugh at them, how colleagues would look down on them, etc. These thoughts might come to dominate and torture their minds, further feeding into the anxiety and making it worse.

Anxiety can also manifest as a feeling or feelings. This might take the form of a general, nebulous, unspecific feeling of dread hanging over them like dark clouds. It may also take a more specific form like a feeling of terror relating to one particular thing. Tension, apprehension, and fear are the most common feelings that people who are experiencing anxiety report. These feelings are partially or entirely irrational but this doesn't lessen its impact in the person suffering from anxiety. Simply knowing that you shouldn't be scared of something doesn't tend to do very much to actually lessen that feeling of fear. Emotions are not always slaves to logic and reason. In fact, quite often it is the opposite.

Finally, anxiety can manifest as behavior. Such behavior can take many forms depending on the nature and severity of the anxiety. Often times the behavior is some type of avoidance. Someone experiencing agoraphobia for example (a fear of open spaces) might avoid going outside. They may realize that they are doing this because of anxiety, or they may not. Some people may convincingly tell themselves all sorts of different reasons why they do the things they do that do not involve admitting to a debilitating problem with anxiety. The key to identifying anxiety manifesting as behavior is to think about the consequences of the actions. Are they interfering with your life? Are they preventing you from functioning in a healthy way? If they are there is something behind those behaviors that is not reason or logic, but likely some disorder such as anxiety, addiction, etc.

The root of anxiety

Regardless of how anxiety manifests or what triggers it, there is a common root cause that accounts for all symptoms of anxiety. Experiencing anxiety is a consequence of a blockage within the body's natural energy system. When the body is in a natural state of energy equilibrium, anxiety is rarely experienced. To the extent that it is, it tends to be a fleeting experience that occurs as a result of a legitimate anxiety-causing stimulus. Over time, our body and brain developed a "fight or flight" response, as explained in detail in the chapter about How EFT Tapping Affects the Brain. In the modern world, we humans fortunately deal with far fewer life or death situations than our ancient ancestors did. Despite this, the "fight or flight" response remains buried deeply in our DNA, impacting our decision making and influencing our reactions. Centuries ago, we needed to keep our guard up much more than we do today. A mistake while foraging for food could mean death at the hands of a hungry predator. The anxiety response was in this sense a pro-social development in humans that encouraged and facilitated our survival. Today though, we don't forage for food, and a startling stimulus is rarely something that could actually harm or kill us. Still though, the body and brain reacts in a way that is similar to the way it would react in a life or death situation. Over time, these false "red alert" type of situations serve to disrupt the flow of energy, altering our thoughts, feelings, and behaviors, in a way that eventually becomes a diagnosable anxiety disorder.

To cure our anxiety we must break through these blockages and restore the natural equilibrium we are intended to have. When the energy flows through our body we will be free of debilitating anxiety disorders and able to do and achieve the things we want in our lives.

Tapping for anxiety

If you struggle with anxiety, the following tapping sequence will bring you some much calm. Begin as always by finding somewhere comfortable to sit, whether in a chair or on the floor. Get comfortable and remember to keep your back straight. Remove any jewelry or glasses that could get in the way.

Get in tune with your body by thinking about the anxiety you are experiencing and rate it on a scale of 1 to 10 with 1 being perfectly comfortable and happy with your mental state and 10 being the maximum state of anxiety. It is important to take this initial benchmark of the level of your anxiety. After the tapping sequence is complete, you will ask yourself this same question again. You will likely experience a 1 or 2 point decrease with each tapping sequence. Often the decrease is more significant than that, such as 3 or 4 points. Sometimes even just a single tapping sequence can reduce your feelings of anxiety by more than 4 points. If you don't notice a change after the initial tapping sequence, you can try going through the entire sequence again from the beginning, or refer to the chapter in this book on what to do if tapping isn't working for you.

I'll reiterate that the more in tune you are with your body before you begin the tapping sequence the more effective tapping can be. Take a moment to review the chapter about what to do before you begin tapping if you need some refreshers on this. Ultimately, remember that *only you* are in control of your body and your mind.

If you would benefit from a visual aid as you proceed through this tapping sequence, remember that I have prepared a free video demonstration for readers of this book. If you think this would be helpful for you, please visit my website at **www.randallawrence.com** to get access to this free video and use it to help you tap through this sequence.

Start by tapping with four fingers on point 1, the side of your hand (or the "karate chop" point). Tap gently. There is no need to be hostile with yourself or hurt yourself. Say out loud:

"Even though I am feeling anxious, I profoundly and completely love and accept myself. I profoundly love and accept the way I feel right now. I profoundly love and accept myself and everything that I am."

Move on to tapping on point 2, your inner wrist. You can tap with two fingers, four fingers, or your opposite wrist. Say out loud:

"Even though I feel this intense anxiety. Even though sometimes I recognize that it makes my life more difficult. Even though sometimes I feel like I will always suffer from anxiety. Even though I feel this way, I profoundly love and accept myself, and my body, and the way it feels right now."

Move on to tapping point 3, the top of your head. Tap with all four fingers on both hands and say out loud:

"I love the way my body feels right now. I know my body responds this way to try to protect me. I know that my feelings of anxiety are my body's way of trying to protect me from harm. I love and accept that my body wants me to be safe from harm. I am profoundly grateful for this reaction. I love and accept every part of my body and I love and accept all of the things it does for me."

Move on to tapping point 4, your eyebrows. You can tap on either side with two fingers. Switch sides when you go through the tapping sequence the second time. Say out loud as you tap:

"I know what it feels like to be calm. To exist in the world without any anxiety clouding my body and mind. I know what it feels like to be at peace. I love and accept that my body wants me to be at peace. Even though I have this anxiety, I know what it feels like to let it go."

Move on to tapping point 5, the side of your eye. Tap with two fingers on either side. When you go through the tapping sequence the second time you can switch sides. Say out loud as you tap:

"I am let go of my anxiety as I move through my blockages and disturbances, releasing myself from the limits it imposes on my life. I know I can do it. I know I can restore my body's naturally peaceful flow of energy."

Move on to tapping point 6, under your eye. Tap with two fingers on either side. When you go through the tapping sequence the second time you can switch sides. Say out loud as you tap:

"I have control over my body. I have control over my emotions. I have control over all of my feelings. I have control over the way my energy flows. I am in control and no one else can control me. I can feel the anxiety fading away. I can feel my energy starting to flow as the blockages and disturbances become smaller and smaller."

Move on to tapping point 7, under your nose. Tap with two fingers and say out loud as you tap:

"This remaining feeling of anxiety is hard to let go of. I understand that my body does not want me to let it go. I understand that my body wants to keep me safe. I know and appreciate all my body does for me. And I've spent so much time believing that I couldn't do it. That I couldn't ever completely rid myself of this anxiety and live a happy life."

Move on to tapping point 8, your chin. Tap with two fingers and say out loud as you tap:

"But now I love and accept that my body responds this way. I profoundly love and accept myself, even with this anxiety. I profoundly love and accept every single part of myself and I know that I am strong enough to let this anxiety go. I know that the love and acceptance I have for myself and my body will give me the strength that I need to live free of anxiety."

Move on to tapping point 9, your collarbone. You can tap on either side with all four fingers. Switch sides when you go through the tapping sequence the second time. Say out loud as you tap:

"I am ready to let go of this remaining anxiety. I do not need this anxiety anymore. I am strong and I will survive and thrive without anxiety. I can feel the anxiety leaving my body. I can feel my strength and commitment to beating this anxiety increasing within me. I know this feeling of strength. I know what it feels like to achieve my goals. I know what it feels like to overcome my challenges and I embrace these feelings within me now."

Move on to tapping point 10, under your arm. Tap on either side with all four fingers. Switch sides when you go through the tapping sequence the second time. Say out loud as you tap:

"I may still some feelings of anxiety within me. I recognize that and I may feel it. But I will not criticize myself for having these feelings. I am choosing to just recognize that they are there and recognize how they feel. And it is OK. I love and accept myself. I love and accept that it is my body trying to protect me. And I love and accept myself enough to let it go."

Take a deep breath in and let it out. Then ask yourself again, on a scale of 1 to 10 how you feel about your anxiety? Do you feel more at peace now? When you think of a situation that might typically induce anxiety within you, do you feel more empowered to take on that situation? Go through the tapping sequence again from the beginning whenever you feel there is some pressure from anxiety that has built up within you and needs to be released.

True tapping miracles: years of anxiety, cured in minutes

Throughout this book I've included a few stories that were told to me by friends, acquaintances, or clients that I have met. I've heard many remarkable stories over the years of the efficacy of EFT tapping and I've selected a small handful to present to you as part of this book. I have personally found these stories to be particularly uplifting and I share them with you in the hopes that they will inspire you on your wellness journey using EFT tapping.

Ron was a client of mine who had a truly sudden and spectacular breakthrough using EFT tapping. His story is an amazing account of the power of tapping to change your life, even when you've suffered for many years. Here is Ron's amazing story:

When I met Ron he was 37 years of age and suffered from a paralyzing fear of water. Ron was not born with this fear, nor did it mysteriously develop over time. Ron recalled the exact moment this fear developed within him. When Ron was a child he had attended a summer camp where he had almost drowned. He was rescued by a camp counselor and was physically unharmed, but from that day on he was deathly scared of water. He hadn't swam in decades since that incident had occurred. His fear went deeper than just swimming however. His anxiety over water was broad and intense. He refused to go the beach because he said even just standing on the sand made him panic and break into a sweat. He felt uncomfortable going to a friend's house who had a swimming pool in the backyard. Even when in the living room of the house, his thoughts would be completely preoccupied with the water-filled pool sitting silently outside the door. Having a bath was out of the question for Ron, and although he knew he had to shower he would do so as quickly and infrequently as possible. Even just washing his hands would sometimes cause a jolt of panic that would distract him from his thoughts.

Ron knew this fear had no real basis in reality. He knew he would never drown in the shower and yet it still terrified him. His intense fear of water interfered with his life daily and he desperately wanted to put it behind him. He had tried a several methods to deal with his anxiety over being in or near water but had not experienced any success.

Based on my conversations with Ron, I believed that EFT tapping could work for him. Ron already had the benefit of knowing exactly where his anxiety was coming from: that one isolated incident as a child at summer camp when he nearly drowned. We talked about how tapping on previous painful memories can eliminate their present day power to influence our thoughts and actions. Ron was basically resigned to living with his anxiety for the rest of his life, but still held out some small hope that something could help him.

We tapped through a session on his anxiety about water and he told me he felt a little better. Not much better, but a little. That was a start, but I told him we should push ahead and see where we got. We got in my car and drove to the beach. As we pulled into the parking lot I cold see Ron visibly perspiring on his forehead. His anxiety was kicking into high-gear as we stopped the car and tapped through another session. This time he said the anxiety dropped 3 points after just one session. We tapped through another and another, dropping his anxiety down further.

I asked Ron to come stand with me on the sand at the beach, something he hadn't done in years. Slowly and with some trepidation, Ron followed me on foot down to the beach. We sat down in the sand and tapped through another session together on Ron's anxiety. Ron couldn't believe it! The anxiety was melting away like an ice cube being blasted by a hair dryer. Without any prompting me from me, Ron stood up and walked towards the water. Standing ankle deep in the lake, Ron turned to me and smiled. I asked how he felt and he said although he still had some residual anxiety, he felt amazing! He had suffered from this anxiety problem for decades, literally since childhood, and in just a few minutes of tapping he felt almost entirely cured!

Ron's story is an inspiring one for people who suffer from any kind of anxiety. Ron was fortunate to cure his anxiety in a matter of minutes. For many, it will take some days or weeks of noticeable progress before a complete cure is achieved. In the grand scheme of things though, whether it takes a few minutes, a few days, or a few weeks, it is an insignificant and trifling amount of time to cure a potentially lifelong debilitating anxiety.

Law of Attraction: how to make more money and attract wealth into your life

I believe that we have the ability, through our thought patterns and our beliefs, to fundamentally change every major aspect of our lives. We are more than merely what exists in the physical world. The limits that are imposed on us and that we impose on ourselves are products of the physical world, of the society that we live in, of the expectations others have for us, etc. They seem like hard limits that define us, but they are not. But they can be shifted. They are not cast in stone.

We all face limiting beliefs in our lives. Many of us are taught throughout our lives that while we may envy the rich or be jealous of the rich, it really is a very bad thing to be wealthy. We are taught this in many ways and absorb this value both consciously and subconsciously. Biblical values like "the meek shall inherit the Earth" and "it is easier for a camel to pass through the eye of a needle than for a rich man to enter heaven" have been handed down over thousands of years. Secular values subtly teach us that money is bad too: we describe wealthy people as "filthy rich" and are taught that "money corrupts". Society teaches us that greed is bad, that having more than you need makes you selfish, etc. There are so many of these limiting beliefs surrounding us from the time we are born that it really shouldn't be a surprise that so many of us adopt these values and let them define the limits of our lives.

We have all been taught that you have to work hard to make money. Maybe this is because the few at the top have a vested interest in having the many at the bottom work hard *for them*. I'm not saying work is not important though, just to be clear. What I am saying is that your mentality and your mindset is far more important than working hard in determining how much or how little wealth you can attract into your life. People tell you that you must work hard to make money, but this only serves to disenfranchise your mentality from your physical labor. You can work yourself to the bone but if you've become the victim of the common limiting beliefs society breeds into us, you will never be wealthy.

What is worse is that not only are so many of us indoctrinated, both consciously and subconsciously, into destructive limiting beliefs about money, but throughout our lives we go on to insidiously pass these same limits on to the people around us. We impose our limiting beliefs on the others just as others have imposed our limiting beliefs us. It is an insidious, parasitic process that plays out largely beneath the threshold of our awareness. Think about the energy of a typical group of people commuting to work on a Monday morning. They are doing what they've come to believe is important, working hard to earn money, and most are not satisfied. Some are down right miserable. They haven't attracted the wealth they want into their lives. Furthermore, they have limiting beliefs telling them being wealthy is an evil thing. It is trivially easy for someone who joins this group to adopt these values. And when these beliefs are widely held in common, they become adopted by virtually all of us as the beliefs of our society.

Modern society is in many ways designed for the majority of us to exist together in a loosely aligned and dissatisfied pack. We go to work, we spend our money, and most of the fruits of our labor go to someone else. Only the very few at the top exist outside of the pack. We make the money, but they get to spend it. This is a system that works just fine for them, and it is one that most of us are stuck in because we do understand the constraints that limit us to this system. We do not understand that the constraints are not external, but internal. The constraints are the beliefs that we have come to adopt based on the values that have been imposed on us. But they are all within us. They are not outside of us. And when we realize this, we empower ourselves. We can knock down these walls because *they are our walls*! They are our own limits that we have imposed on ourselves and that we can learn to stop imposing on ourselves. When you come to realize that the other end of the leash around your neck is in your own hand and not someone else's, you can take yourself in whatever direction you want.

How to break through negative limiting beliefs

If you understand everything I've laid down above regarding our negative limiting beliefs being internal to us, the next obvious question is how do we break through these negative beliefs? Certainly understanding where limiting beliefs come from, how we adopt them, and how they serve to hold us back from attracting the wealth we want and deserve into our lives is the first step. But it is not enough to just understand this. We need to go further and take proactive steps to break free of these chains that are holding us down.

As I've explained throughout this book, EFT tapping is a remarkable technique that can be applied to successfully break through energy blockages and restore the natural equilibrium we are all born with. When you apply the techniques taught in this book you can make dramatic, fundamental changes in virtually every aspect of your life. Breaking through energy blockages is much the same as breaking through limiting beliefs. The blockages in our energy fields and pathways cripple us in the same way that limiting beliefs do. This is why EFT tapping can successfully be applied to destroy not only our energy blockages, but also our limiting beliefs.

Let's tap through our limiting beliefs about money that are preventing us from attracting real wealth into our lives. Begin as always by finding a comfortable seated position, spine straight, not slouching or laying down. Clear your mind and begin to focus on your financial situation as it is currently and as it has been in the past. On a scale of 1 to 10, how do you feel about your ability to attract wealth into your life? A 1 is the lowest level, complete dissatisfaction and despair about your ability to attract wealth into your life. A 10 is the highest level, complete satisfaction about your ability to attract wealth into your life.

If you would benefit from a visual aid as you proceed through this tapping sequence, remember that I have prepared a free video demonstration for readers of this book. If you think this would be helpful for you, please visit my website at **www.randallawrence.com** to get access to this free video and use it to help you tap through this sequence.

Now begin the tapping session by tapping with four fingers on point 1, the side of the hand (or the "karate chop point"). Tap gently. There is no need to be aggressive with yourself or hurt yourself. Say out loud:

"even though I am feeling so dissatisfied with my ability to attract wealth into my life right now, I profoundly and completely love and accept myself. I profoundly love and accept the way I feel right now. I profoundly love and accept myself and everything that I am."

Move on to tapping on point 2, the inner wrist. You can tap with two fingers, four fingers, or your opposite wrist. Say out loud:

"Even though I feel so dissatisfied with my ability to attract wealth into my life. Even though sometimes I feel so unable to change my financial situation. Even though sometimes I feel like I will never have the wealth in my life that I want and deserve. Even though I feel this way, I profoundly love and accept myself and the way I feel right now."

Move on to tapping point 3, the top of the head. Tap with all four fingers on both hands and say out loud:

"I love the way my body and mind feel right now. I know my body and mind respond in this way to try to protect me. I know this I have been raised in a world full of limiting beliefs that have been imposed on me. I love and accept that I am not at fault for adopting these limiting beliefs as my own. I know it is not my fault and I love and accept every part of my body and mind and I love and accept all of the things they do for me."

Move on to tapping point 4, the eyebrows. You can tap on either side with two fingers. Switch sides when you go through the tapping sequence the second time. Say out loud as you tap:

"I can imagine what it would feel like to attract an abundance of wealth into my life. I know what it feels like to be completely satisfied, without any worries or concerns about money. I know what it feels like to be at peace with myself and the world. Even though I know I have these limiting beliefs inside of me, I know what it feels like to break through these limits."

Move on to tapping point 5, side of the eye. Tap with two fingers on either side. When you go through the tapping sequence the second time you can switch sides. Say out loud as you tap:

"I am open to feeling free of these limits as I move through my blockages, releasing all of these negative beliefs that have held me back. Embracing potential. Embracing limitlessness. Embracing my body's natural desire and ability to attract the wealth that I want and deserve."

Move on to tapping point 6, under the eye. Tap with two fingers on either side. When you go through the tapping sequence the second time you can switch sides. Say out loud as you tap:

"I have control over the things I attract into my life. I have control over my beliefs. I have control over all of my limits. I have control over the way my energy flows. I am in control and no one else can control me. I can feel the limiting beliefs about money starting to leave my body. I can feel my energy starting to flow as the blockages and disturbances become smaller and smaller."

Move on to tapping point 7, under the nose. Tap with two fingers and say out loud as you tap:

"These remaining limiting beliefs in my body and mind are hard to let go of. I understand that my body and mind do not want me to let it go. I understand that my body and mind want to cling to the familiar and they want to keep these beliefs even though they are negative and destructive. My body wants to keep me safe. My body wants to protect me. And I've spent so much time trying to ignore my own negativity, or pretend it isn't there."

Move on to tapping point 8, the chin. Tap with two fingers and say out loud as you tap:

"But now I love and accept that my body responds this way. I profoundly love and accept myself, even with these limiting beliefs that prevent me from attracting the wealth I want and deserve. I profoundly love and accept every single part of myself even with all of these negative beliefs. And although I am now ready to let go of these beliefs, I know that even if I don't let them go that I still completely love and accept every part of myself."

Move on to tapping point 9, the collarbone. You can tap on either side with all four fingers. Switch sides when you go through the tapping sequence the second time. Say out loud as you tap:

"But I am ready to let go of these remaining beliefs that limit me. I do not need them anymore. I can feel them leaving my body and I can feel the calm and peace coming into my body. I know this feeling of peacefulness. I know this feeling of calm. And I embrace these feelings within me now."

Move on to tapping point 10, under your arm. Tap on either side with all four fingers. Switch sides when you go through the tapping sequence the second time. Say out loud as you tap:

"I may still have some negative limiting beliefs inside me, and I may still feel them holding me back sometimes. I recognize this and I may feel this. But I will not criticize myself for having these beliefs. It is not my fault. I am choosing to just recognize that they are there and recognize how they feel. And it is OK. I love and accept myself even with all of these limiting beliefs. I love and accept that it is my body and mind trying to protect me. And I love and accept myself enough to let them go."

You will probably want to go through these tapping script at least twice. After you have finished, ask yourself on a scale of 1 to 10 how are you feeling right now about your negative limiting beliefs about money and your ability to attract wealth into your life? Feel empowered and break through your limiting beliefs so you can attract all of the wealth you want and deserve into your life!

Law of Attraction: fall in love, improve your relationships, and attract the people you want into your life

When we are in a state of love and joy, we are in a more attractive state. We will attract more love and more joy into our lives when we are already existing in this state and projecting it outwards to others. Attraction is something that feeds into itself in this sense. This is a good reason why you should adopt as your own personal mission, to live a life of love and happiness for yourself and for those around you.

We can attract the people we need and want into our lives. Sometimes this will be someone similar to us, but other times it will be someone who is our opposite: the yin to our yang. For example if you are the type of person who is more introverted and not very outgoing, you may find it beneficial to attract into your life someone who is more extroverted. As an introvert, having an extrovert for a partner can open up a side of social and interpersonal relationships that you may not otherwise have access to. Similarly, an introvert may help to develop within an extroverted partner an appreciation of themselves, of the moment, of the pleasures of life apart from group socialization. This is a method of growth and it we can sometimes best self-actualize by attracting opposites into our lives. It is important to keep this in mind as you go about thinking of the type of person you want to attract into your life. You may think you want someone just like yourself, but in fact, this may not be the ideal situation for you.

Love is perhaps the richest emotion and experience that we can access as humans. There are various layers or qualities of love. Sometimes love can take the form of generosity or giving. It can also take the form of peacefulness and acceptance, of yourself, your partner, and the world at large. It can take the form of energy, excitement, and attraction. It can take the form of sexuality. Love is amazingly deep and complex but at its highest and purest form, it is unconditional. It does not depend on anything outside itself and there are no contingencies. It simple exists as a rock through time, unchanged, unaffected, forever pure. For me, the highest purpose and benefit of relationships is to experience this pure love. We must strive to give this pure, unconditional love to those around us, for only when we project it outwards can we expect it to come back to us.

The world is a mirror, of sorts. If we project our purest and most sincere love and happiness outward to the world, we will find that the world reflects this back upon us. And if instead we project our selfishness, and our insecurities, and whatever other negativity we have lurking within us, we will find that the world reflects this negativity right back at us. We attract the things we feel, believe, and project into the world, for better or for worse.

Attracting a specific person

Whenever I talk about the law of attraction as applied to love and relationships and facilitated through EFT tapping I am frequently asked how to go about attracting a specific person. Lots of people have a sense that they want a particular person in their lives and don't know quite how to go about making that happen. Sometimes this person is an acquaintance or even a stranger. But the person seeking to attract them into their lives feels that this other person would be perfect for them. They could have a great romantic relationship together, if only they could get together somehow. Sometimes I am asked this question about an ex-partner and how they could be attracted *back* into the person's life; how they could rekindle the romantic relationship they once had.

The first thing I have to say about this topic is that we all have our own freewill. The law of attraction should not be viewed as something that can be used to dominate and compel others against their will. We can not simply force someone to be in our lives if they themselves do not want to be. The law of attraction as it applies to relationships is about projecting outward what you want to attract back towards yourself. When you think about the pleasant feelings you have associated with the particular person you want to attract, you need to focus on these positive feelings and project them outward. You need to do this because if the other person feels what you are feeling, they will want the same thing as you! You need them to feel this way too. The fact is though, is that you can't target your projection only towards one person and no one else. We are what we are, we feel what we feel, and this is what we project. Projections are not selective just as the mirror is not selective when you look in to it. The mirror shows you for you, all the good and all the bad, and it shows it to whoever is looking at the mirror. When you project love and joy therefore, you are not projecting it at an individual, but rather at the world at large. If you want to attract a specific person, you might see this as a disadvantage. I encourage you not to see it this way. The fact is that you while you may not attract the person you think you want into your life, you will attract the *person that is right for you* based on your projections. This is actually much better and more powerful than merely targeting a single person. When you seek to attract love and joy and positivity into your life by projecting these things outward, you will get them back in some form. Do not be closed off to how they come to you and do not limit yourself only to what you think you want.

Tapping for love and attraction

You cannot expect to project anything close to pure love and joy into the world if your body's naturally energy is flowing freely and vigorously throughout you as it is meant to. The more blockages you have in your energy field and pathways the less positivity you can radiate to the outside world. In order to activate the law of attraction to attract love into your life therefore, you must facilitate your own love, joy, and happiness by tapping through your blockages.

To tap through these blockages and activate the law of attraction, you need to think about the things that are holding you back. Sometimes the blockages may not be immediately obvious. I remember a client telling me how he longed for a fulfilling relationship and was ready to attract this into his life. He couldn't see any reason why this hadn't happened. The fact was though, that he was full of negativity and selfishness. He wanted a relationship to fulfill his own needs. He wanted someone that looked nice who would hang off his arm at social events, prepare meals for him, listen to him and be there for him. He wanted a relationship because he wanted it to benefit *him.* And this is exactly what he project into the world. Not love, or joy, or happiness, but selfishness. Wanting love in your life is very different from *feeling and projecting love outside of yourself.* You need to think carefully about what it is you are projecting because this is what dictates what you will attract.

Once you have a sense of the negativity and blockages inside you and what you may be projecting outwardly, find a comfortable place to sit. As always, sit with your spine straight and take notice of your body and your surroundings. Ask yourself on a scale of 1 to 10 to rate the intensity of impediments to projecting pure love. A 1 on this scale would be no impediment: you are projecting pure love and joy out to the world. A 10 on this scale would be a maximum impediment: you are projecting only negativity, such as your own selfishness out to the world.

If you would benefit from a visual aid as you proceed through this tapping sequence, remember that I have prepared a free video demonstration for readers of this book. If you think this would be helpful for you, please visit my website at **www.randallawrence.com** to get access to this free video and use it to help you tap through this sequence.

When you are ready, begin the tapping sequence. Start by tapping with four fingers on point 1, the side of the hand (or the "karate chop point"). Tap gently. There is no need to be aggressive with yourself or hurt yourself. Say out loud:

"even though I am feeling this negativity inside me right now, I profoundly and completely love and accept myself. I profoundly love and accept who I am as a person. I profoundly love and accept myself and everything that I am."

Move on to tapping on point 2, the inner wrist. You can tap with two fingers, four fingers, or your opposite wrist. Say out loud:

"Even though I feel this negativity and selfishness inside me. Even though I know that I do not yet feel pure love. Even though sometimes I feel like I will never feel and project pure love and joy into the world. Even though I feel this way, I profoundly love and accept myself, and my body, and the way it feels right now."

Move on to tapping point 3, the top of the head. Tap with all four fingers on both hands and say out loud:

"I love the way my body feels right now. I know my body responds this way to try to protect me. I know that being selfish is my body's natural reaction to try to get the thing I want in life. I love and accept that my body wants the best for me. I am profoundly grateful for this reaction. I love and accept every part of my body and I love and accept all of the things it does for me."

Move on to tapping point 4, the eyebrows. You can tap on either side with two fingers. Switch sides when you go through the tapping sequence the second time. Say out loud as you tap:

"I know what it feels like to be loving. I know what it feels like to be completely selfless, without any negativity holding me back. I love and accept that my body wants the best for me, even though it is sometimes counterproductive in what it causes me to feel and project."

Move on to tapping point 5, side of the eye. Tap with two fingers on either side. When you go through the tapping sequence the second time you can switch sides. Say out loud as you tap:

"I am open to feeling pure selfless love and joy as I move through my blockages and disturbances, releasing all of this negativity that has built up within me. Embracing love. Embracing joy. Embracing my body's naturally peaceful flow of energy."

Move on to tapping point 6, under the eye. Tap with two fingers on either side. When you go through the tapping sequence the second time you can switch sides. Say out loud as you tap:

"I have control over my body. I have control over my emotions. I have control over all of my feelings. I have control over the way my energy flows. I am in control and no one else can control me. I can feel the negativity starting to leave my body. I can feel the love starting to grow within me and my energy flow as the blockages and disturbances become smaller and smaller."

Move on to tapping point 7, under the nose. Tap with two fingers and say out loud as you tap:

"This remaining negativity in my body is hard to let go of. I understand that my body does not want me to let it go. I understand that my body wants to keep it. My body wants to keep me safe. My body wants to protect me. But I know that now is the time to embrace positivity."

Move on to tapping point 8, the chin. Tap with two fingers and say out loud as you tap:

"And although I love and accept that my body responds this way, and I profoundly love and accept myself, even with this negativity, I know now is the time to let it go. I profoundly love and accept every single part of myself and the world. And although I am now ready to let go any remaining negativity, I know that even if I don't let it go that I still completely love and accept every part of myself."

Move on to tapping point 9, the collarbone. You can tap on either side with all four fingers. Switch sides when you go through the tapping sequence the second time. Say out loud as you tap:

"But I am ready to let go of this remaining negativity that I am projecting into the world. I do not need it anymore. I do not need to be selfish. I can feel the negativity leaving my body and I can feel the love and joy coming into my body. I know this feeling of love. I know this feeling of joy. And I embrace these feelings within me now."

Move on to tapping point 10, under your arm. Tap on either side with all four fingers. Switch sides when you go through the tapping sequence the second time. Say out loud as you tap:

"I may still feel selfishness and negativity from time to time. I recognize it and I may feel it. But I will not criticize myself for having these feelings. I am choosing to just recognize that they are there and recognize how they feel. And it is OK. I love and accept myself and the world. And I love and accept myself enough to embrace pure love."

Once you have gone through the tapping sequence twice, take a moment and evaluate your feelings again on the 1 to 10 scale. How do you feel about your impediments to pure love? What do you think you are projecting into the world? Remember, that in order to attract the love and life you want, you need to remove the negative blockages that are negatively impacting your outward projections. Continue to tap through these blockages as you move closer and closer to projecting pure love and joy to the world.

True tapping miracles: The young family man headed for divorce

Throughout this book I've included a few stories that were told to me by friends, acquaintances, or clients that I have met. I've heard many remarkable stories over the years of the efficacy of EFT tapping and I've selected a small handful to present to you as part of this book. I have personally found these stories to be particularly uplifting and I share them with you in the hopes that they will inspire you on your wellness journey using EFT tapping.

When I was at a conference on energy psychology a few years ago, one of the attendees approached me and told me about his experience using EFT tapping to save his marriage. I asked him if he would be willing to share his story with the readers of my upcoming book and he agreed. The following is his story, in his own words:

I was 34 years old when I first heard about tapping. I was at a friend's cottage on Memorial Day and over a beer and some barbecue I confided to him that my marriage was rapidly falling apart. My wife Natasha and I had been married for only three years at that point and we were barely on speaking terms. I had been sleeping on the couch for weeks. The only time I would sleep in our bed is when she would go away with "friends" for the weekend. She never told me she was having an affair and I never asked. I guess I just didn't want to hear her confirm what I already knew. We were more emotionally distant than ever before and it felt like it was just a matter of time before we would each be hiring a divorce lawyer. I remember sharing all of this personal hurt with my friend Taylor that day and as the sun went down over the lake behind the cottage, he introduced me to "tapping".

I had never heard of tapping before this, but Taylor raved about it. He said he had been through some difficult times with his wife and he had used tapping to help him get through with his marriage intact. He told me how he shared tapping with his wife and together they would tap through their emotional distress, working together to heal their marriage. I wasn't sure what to make of this. On the one hand, I trusted that Taylor was being honest with me and that tapping had really worked well for him and his wife. On the other hand, it sounded a little bit crazy! How is tapping on certain points on my face and body supposed to fix my marriage?! It just didn't make sense to me. I was naive and ignorant about the power of tapping. When I left Taylor's cottage the next day I had already practically forgotten about it.

Two months after that Memorial Day weekend, my daughter turned 2 years old. Natasha and I could barely stand to be in the same room as we tried to celebrate her birthday and pretend things were OK. But they weren't OK. They were terrible and I was a wreck. I was desperate. Taylor and his wife were at our house for our small celebration and seeing the two of them looking so happy and so in love made me think of all the good times Natasha and I had shared together. I also remembered that Memorial Day weekend when Taylor and I sat out on his deck and he told me what tapping had done for him and his marriage. That is when I decided to take the plunge.

Later that evening after we had all eaten, I lured Taylor out to the garage under the pretext of checking something on the car. Once we were alone in the garage I asked him for help. I asked him to show me how tapping worked. I was ready to earnestly and humbly open my mind to tapping in the hope that I might find some emotional calm, some peace of mind, and maybe even a fix for my badly broken marriage. Standing out there in the garage that evening, under the single incandescent bulb burning above our heads, Taylor took me through me very first tapping session. I was surprised when within minutes I felt my stress level drop from a 9 out of 10, down to a 7 out of 10. Could tapping really be so effective? I remember falling asleep that night, still on the couch, but excited for the first time in months that there may actually be a solution to my marriage difficulties.

Over the next month I tapped at least twice a day, but often more like four or five times. I introduced tapping to Natasha and after a bit of coaxing I successfully convinced her to try it. She was as surprised as I was when she saw the power of tapping! We both knew that although we had many hostile feelings toward each other at the time, we wanted to have the great relationship we had before. We didn't want to get a divorce. We wanted to be together in a happy marriage and happy family, raising our daughter together. We committed to using tapping as the tool that would bring us together again. For us, finding tapping was like a surgeon finding the scalpel that he needs to cut out and remove some cancerous growth from a body. We read more and more about tapping, improving our ability to use our new tool effectively. Together we used EFT tapping to cut out our deepest emotional blockages, healing our marriage, our family, and each other.

Today, two years later, Natasha and I have never been happier. Our daughter is starting kindergarten and Natasha just gave birth to our second child, a boy! We are both so thankful for having discovered tapping when we did, before it was too late.

EFT Tapping for rejection and heartbreak

Rejection and heartbreak are some of the most emotionally devastating types of pain. The pain is very real. Part of the reason why the pain can be so great is because we are reopening old wounds. As infants and as children we all experienced times where we were rejected, ignored, or somehow didn't receive what we needed from our primary caregivers. Whether we can actually remember incidents like this or not, they have happened to all of us at some point and are buried deep in our subconscious. When emotionally painful things happened to us in our early years of life, they never went away. They may have healed in the way that a scab heals over a cut, but the wound is still there, ready to have the scab ripped away and hurt us again as adults.

Another reason why rejection and heartbreak can be so painful is it reinforces our own beliefs of inadequacy. Virtually all of us feel inadequate in some way. We have insecurities about our skills, or our abilities, uncertainties about interpersonal relationships, and feelings that we simply aren't good enough not only according to the standards set by others, but even according to *our own standards*.

We can't just ignore these hurtful feelings. Feelings do not go away when they are ignored. They continue to thrive below the surface of our subconscious, adversely affecting our well-being, and impacting our disposition daily.

Rather than ignore what is hurting us and holding us back, we must face these things head on. We must acknowledge what they are and develop a plan of attack to break through them. As explained above, the pain stemming from a breakup is often linked to some prior pain. Some bad memory of another time we were rejected as a child. Often times, this prior pain is the real driver of the present day pain. As adults, we are far less vulnerable than children. We are autonomous, powerful, and have much more in our lives than children do. But when we are rejected as adults, it brings back to us the intense feelings of helplessness and abandonment we all experienced at least a few times as a child. That sharp feeling of being unwanted cuts into us just as deeply now as it did back then. To deal with the present pain, we need to acknowledge that the present day pain and the present day breakup is only the tip of the iceberg. It is our life experience and prior pain that is being triggered and is suddenly deployed as a barrier within our energy flow, throwing off our equilibrium and scattering the pieces of our lives. We need to target these blockages and tap through them so that we can gather our thoughts and emotions and move on with our lives.

Here is a great tapping script to use after a breakup. Remember that you can improve upon it yourself by referring to the chapter in this book about how to target your own tapping and create your own tapping script. The more you can drill down on the exact source of your pain, the more successfully you can apply EFT tapping as therapy to ease the intense heartbreak you may be experiencing.

Now let's prepare to start the tapping sequence. Sit in a comfortable position with your back straight. Take a moment to notice your body and the environment surrounding you. You can review the chapter on preparing to tap if you need a refresher. On a scale of 1 to 10 rate the intensity of the heartbreak you are feeling right now, where 1 is only a very mild feeling, and 10 is the maximum most devastating heartbreak possible.

If you would benefit from a visual aid as you proceed through this tapping sequence, remember that I have prepared a free video demonstration for readers of this book. If you think this would be helpful for you, please visit my website at **www.randallawrence.com** to get access to this free video and use it to help you tap through this sequence.

When you are ready to begin, start by tapping with four fingers on point 1, the side of the hand (or the "karate chop point"). Tap gently. There is no need to be aggressive with yourself or hurt yourself. Say out loud:

"even though I am feeling this intense heartbreak right now, I profoundly and completely love and accept myself. I profoundly love and accept the way I feel right now. I profoundly love and accept myself and everything that I am."

Move on to tapping on point 2, the inner wrist. You can tap with two fingers, four fingers, or your opposite wrist. Say out loud:

"Even though I feel so much pain right now. Even though I feel like I am unwanted and unloved. Even though I feel like my whole world has been blown up and I will never recover from this. Even though I feel this way, I profoundly love and accept myself, and my body, and the way it feels right now."

Move on to tapping point 3, the top of the head. Tap with all four fingers on both hands and say out loud:

"**I love the way my body feels right now. I know my body responds this way to try to protect me. I know this is my body's reaction based on the experiences I have had throughout my life and I love and accept that my body wants me to be safe from harm. I am profoundly grateful for this reaction. I love and accept every part of my body and I love and accept all of the things it does for me.**"

Move on to tapping point 4, the eyebrows. You can tap on either side with two fingers. Switch sides when you go through the tapping sequence the second time. Say out loud as you tap:

"**I know what it feels like to be loved. I know what it feels like to be completely happy in a relationship, without any worries in the world. I love and accept that my body wants to protect me from harm so that I may return to a peaceful state of happiness and contentment. Even though I feel so heartbroken right now, I know what love feels like.**"

Move on to tapping point 5, side of the eye. Tap with two fingers on either side. When you go through the tapping sequence the second time you can switch sides. Say out loud as you tap:

"**I am open to feeling love and happiness as I move through my blockages and disturbances, releasing all of these intense emotions that have built up within me. Embracing peace. Embracing love. Embracing my body's natural flow of energy.**"

Move on to tapping point 6, under the eye. Tap with two fingers on either side. When you go through the tapping sequence the second time you can switch sides. Say out loud as you tap:

"I have control over my body. I have control over my emotions. I have control over all of my feelings. I have control over the way my energy flows. I am in control and no one else can control me. I can feel the pain and despair starting to leave my body. I can feel my energy starting to flow as the blockages and disturbances become smaller and smaller."

Move on to tapping point 7, under the nose. Tap with two fingers and say out loud as you tap:

"This remaining pain and feelings of abandonment in my body are hard to let go of. I understand that my body does not want me to let it go. I understand that my body wants to keep it. My body wants to keep me safe. My body wants to protect me. My body doesn't want me to be hurt again, and I appreciate that my body is trying to protect me."

Move on to tapping point 8, the chin. Tap with two fingers and say out loud as you tap:

"I love and accept that my body responds this way. I profoundly love and accept myself, even with these overwhelming painful emotions. I profoundly love and accept every single part of myself even with all of this heartbreak. And although I am now ready to let it go, I know that even if I don't let it go that I still completely love and accept every part of myself."

Move on to tapping point 9, the collarbone. You can tap on either side with all four fingers. Switch sides when you go through the tapping sequence the second time. Say out loud as you tap:

"But I am ready to let go of this remaining pain that I am feeling right now. I do not need this heartbreak anymore. I can live and be strong without it. I can feel it leaving my body and I can feel the love and acceptance coming into my body. I know this feeling of love. I know this feeling of acceptance. And I embrace these feelings within me now."

Move on to tapping point 10, under your arm. Tap on either side with all four fingers. Switch sides when you go through the tapping sequence the second time. Say out loud as you tap:

"I may still feel unwanted, and heartbroken, and abandoned. I recognize these emotions and I may feel them. But I will not criticize myself for having these feelings. I am choosing to just recognize that they are there and recognize how they feel. And it is OK. I love and accept myself despite this breakup. I love and accept that my feelings of heartbreak is my body trying to protect me. And I love and accept myself enough to let it go."

If this was the first time you have tapped through this script, go back to the beginning and tap through a second time. Once you've tapped on your heartbreak twice through the above script (or your own script modified according to the instructions in this book) rate your feeling of heartbreak again on a scale of 1 to 10. Many clients I've worked with in coaching sessions report a drop of 3, 4, or even 5 points. Tapping on heartbreak can be a very effective way to make the emotional pain subside, however it is typical that the devastating feelings will slowly build in intensity again. If they do, just tap through them again as needed. You will find each time they come back they get less and less intense until eventually your blockages are cleared completely, your equilibrium is restored, and your broken heart is completely repaired.

True tapping miracles: The devastating breakup

Throughout this book I've included a few stories that were told to me by friends, acquaintances, or clients that I have met. I've heard many remarkable stories over the years of the efficacy of EFT tapping and I've selected a small handful to present to you as part of this book. I have personally found these stories to be particularly uplifting and I share them with you in the hopes that they will inspire you on your wellness journey using EFT tapping.

Last year one of my younger readers reached out to me and shared the following amazing story of how she used EFT tapping to recover from a breakup that had devastated her. I asked her if she would be willing to share her story with the readers of my upcoming book and she agreed. The following is her story, in her own words:

When I was 24 years old I went through a devastating breakup with my boyfriend Daryl. We were both still young at the time but we had been together for 7 years, since we were both in high school. He was the only serious boyfriend I had ever had in my life and I was sure he was "the one". We were so perfect for each other that even back in high school our friends would joke with us, asking why we didn't just go ahead and get married already. I always assumed that is exactly what would happen when the time was right. Boy was I wrong.

I still vividly remember the night I discovered he had been cheating on me. He was in the shower and I was sitting on his bed. We were going out for dinner that night and I was going to bring up how I thought we should start seriously thinking about moving in together. We had talked about it previously but the time never seemed right for various reasons. I realize now he was just making excuses.

Anyway, while Daryl was in the shower his cell phone went off on the nightstand beside the bed. I looked over and saw it was a text message. I wasn't trying to snoop, I really wasn't. But we were supposed to meet up with some of his friends after dinner and I thought it might be one of them, notifying us about a change of plans or something, so I picked up the phone and read the incoming text message: "can't stop thinking about you after last night babe xoxo see you Sunday". My heart skipped a beat. It must be some kind of mistake. Surely this person had the wrong number or something. But the phone number was in Daryl's contact list. "Bree". I was unable to hold back from violating his privacy as I started scrolling through previous texts between Bree and the love of my life. There were lots of messages. Lots and lots and lots of messages, going back over three months. I felt sick, and angry, and sad all at once. I never suspected anything and this sudden realization hit me like a sack of bricks.

By the time Daryl finished his shower I was a mess. Tears were streaming down my face and my hands were shaking.
"What's wrong?" Daryl asked when he saw me sitting there in obvious distress.
"Who is Bree?" I trembled, not even sure why I was asking a question I didn't want to know the answer to. The color ran out of Daryl's face. He knew he was caught.

"She's... a friend... from work," he replied with obvious uncertainty in his voice. I swore at him as I ran out to my car, crying all the way home.

The days that followed were the darkest of my adult life. Never had I felt so rejected and heartbroken. My confidence and feelings of self-worth had totally evaporated when I read that text messages and I wasn't sure I would ever get them back. I sat alone in my dark room. I couldn't eat, I couldn't think, I couldn't do anything. I'd try to watch TV or listen to music but everything would just remind me of Daryl.

Days turned to weeks and weeks to months. I managed to control the crying but inside I was still a wreck. I felt like I couldn't fully pay attention to anything. Like I was never really present in the moment anymore. Barely an hour could go by without me thinking of him. It was hell. My dad suggested I see a psychologist and I tried a few sessions but his "talk therapy" only made things worse as I would just dwell that much more on how devastating the whole thing was to me.

I knew I needed help from someone, but I didn't know who or what. I started Googling for alternatives to traditional talk therapy and eventually I stumbled across something called "EFT tapping". I had never heard of tapping before but it sounded easy to try, and I liked that it didn't involve rehashing all of my hurt feelings with a stranger. I tried tapping using a generic tapping script I found about stress and I was surprised that I actually felt a bit better afterwards. I certainly didn't feel I was back to my old self yet, but it was encouraging that I felt even a slight improvement.

The next day I ordered some books online in the hopes that if I could learn more about tapping and get better at it, I might be able to employ this strategy more effectively. For the first time since I read that devastating text message, I felt like there might finally be some light at the end of the tunnel.

I continued tapping over the weeks and months that followed, writing and using my own tapping scripts as I went. I learned everything I could about this fascinating therapy and was encouraged by the increasingly positive results it delivered. I would still have sudden moments where I would feel emotionally overwhelmed by what had happened and be on the verge of tears, but I knew that whenever that happened I could just retreat to a quiet corner somewhere, tap through it, and five minutes later I would be feeling fine again.

Eventually, thanks to EFT tapping, I finally got over Daryl. When I think about him now I can appreciate the good times we had together and be thankful for them, while not holding any resentment or ill-will towards him for what happened. In the end, things just didn't work out for us and that is fine. In fact, I'm actually grateful for what happened because without that horrible experience I may never have found EFT tapping.

Today, not only do I use tapping to work through my daily stresses and problems, but I have also taught this remarkable therapy to friends who have seen amazing success with it as well. And as for my love life? Well, once I was over Daryl I stopped tapping to get over my heartbreak and started tapping to attract a new and more compatible partner. My current boyfriend Nathan and I have been together for six months now and things are going very well between us. I have honestly never been happier in my entire life.

EFT tapping for pain relief

One of the most surprising applications of EFT tapping has been in the area of pain relief. Looking at the history of EFT tapping and its treatment by the scientific community, it is apparent that while the psychological benefits of EFT were more readily accepted, the idea that this therapeutic technique could reduce physical pain was met with a heightened skepticism by scientists and doctors. It is one thing to change your habits, thoughts, and emotions, they reasoned, but quite another to reduce pain within the body. It is always somewhat astounding to me when an amazing, easy, accessible, and free technique like tapping is met with scorn by the medical and scientific community. This, after all, is the same community that too often would sooner write out a prescription for Oxycontin/paracetamol or some other addictive cocktail of industrial strength drugs that aim to mask the symptoms while ignoring the underlying condition. Unfortunately, many educated and well meaning professionals have been ground up by the machinery of the pharmaceutical industry and come out the other end believing and repeating the dogma that this very rich and powerful industry seeks to indoctrinate them with. It isn't that prescription medication is always bad. For many people it is a legitimate need that enhances or even saves their lives. The problem is that nowadays drugs are seen as a panacea. They have become plan A, instead of plan B or C. They have become ubiquitous and omnipresent and marketed to "cure" virtually anything whether it is a legitimate condition or not. Further, in many cases the side effects of the drugs are themselves worse than the original condition. From what I have seen I believe this is a global issue, although in Europe the pharmaceutical industry seems to be kept more in check by government than here in the United States where it sometimes seems as though these massive private corporations have simply subsumed control of the Food and Drug Administration. I believe it is these private financial interests that have accounted for a historical suspicion and dismissal of legitimate therapy like EFT tapping and many others.

At the present time however, the evidence is becoming undeniable to even hardened advocates of the old school of thought driven by the pharmaceutical industry. EFT tapping can be a safe and effective way to relieve all kinds of different pain. It is not appropriate for everything and I am certainly not encouraging it's use as a substitute for professional medical care or advice. Nothing is lost however by tapping in conjunction with other treatments. I have met enough people who told me their stories of how tapping worked when nothing else would that I am convinced of its efficacy, even aside from the increasing scientific acceptance EFT tapping is presently gaining.

The reason why EFT tapping can provide effective pain relief is actually quite simple for someone who understands energy physiology. In our natural state, energy flows freely throughout the body according to the natural pathways without anything to get in its way. This is our equilibrium: our ideal state of existence. Throughout life however, our energy pathways can become blocked by all kinds of things we may encounter in life. When we face adversity or difficulty, one impact it may have on our body is to reduce the proper flow of energy through a particular pathway. When our energy flow becomes inhibited and our chakras clogged, this can manifest as a physical consequence. It could manifest as a lack of energy and a general feeling of fatigue. It could take myriad psychological or habitual consequence as explained throughout this book. Or it could manifest as pain in a particular spot in the body, such as a joint or a muscle. When pain occurs in this way, tapping through the blockages and restoring the body's natural energy equilibrium can bring immediate and dramatic pain relief that is more effective than any drug, and without any of the nasty side effects!

If you are suffering from physical pain, you may find the following tapping sequence brings you relief. Sit in a comfortable spot with your back straight. Depending on the type of pain you are experiencing it may not be possible to get entirely comfortable, which is fine. Just do your best. Clear your mind and focus on your body, the pain, and its intensity. Rate the pain on a scale of 1 to 10, where 1 is a very low level of pain and 10 is the maximum possible level of pain.

If you would benefit from a visual aid as you proceed through this tapping sequence, remember that I have prepared a free video demonstration for readers of this book. If you think this would be helpful for you, please visit my website at **www.randallawrence.com** to get access to this free video and use it to help you tap through this sequence.

Start the tapping sequence by tapping with four fingers on point 1, the side of the hand (or the "karate chop point"). Tap gently. There is no need to be aggressive with yourself or hurt yourself. Say out loud:

"even though I am feeling so much pain in my body right now, I profoundly and completely love and accept myself. I profoundly love and accept the way I feel right now. I profoundly love and accept myself and everything that I am."

Move on to tapping on point 2, the inner wrist. You can tap with two fingers, four fingers, or your opposite wrist. Say out loud:

"Even though I feel so much pain in my body right now right now. Even though sometimes the pain feels overwhelming. Even though sometimes I feel like I can't focus on anything or function the way I want to because of this intense pain. Even though I feel this way, I profoundly love and accept myself, and my body, and the way it feels right now."

Move on to tapping point 3, the top of the head. Tap with all four fingers on both hands and say out loud:

"I love the way my body feels right now. I love my body and all that it does for me. I know this pain I am feeling is not my fault. And it is not my body's fault. My body works so well in so many ways and I am profoundly grateful for everything my body does for me. I love and accept every part of my body and I love and accept all of the things it does for me."

Move on to tapping point 4, the eyebrows. You can tap on either side with two fingers. Switch sides when you go through the tapping sequence the second time. Say out loud as you tap:

"I know what it feels like to be free of pain. My body has been free of pain before and it can be free of pain again. My body can return to this peaceful feeling, free of any pain. Even though I have so much pain right now, I know what it feels like to be free of pain."

Move on to tapping point 5, side of the eye. Tap with two fingers on either side. When you go through the tapping sequence the second time you can switch sides. Say out loud as you tap:

"I am open to letting go of the pain as I move through my blockages and disturbances, releasing all of this intense pain that exists in my body. Embracing calmness. Embracing peacefulness. Embracing my body's naturally peaceful flow of energy."

Move on to tapping point 6, under the eye. Tap with two fingers on either side. When you go through the tapping sequence the second time you can switch sides. Say out loud as you tap:

"I have control over my body. I have control over my emotions. I have control over all of my feelings. I have control over the way my energy flows. I am in control and no one else can control me. I can feel the pain starting to leave my body. I can feel my energy starting to flow as the blockages and disturbances become smaller and smaller."

Move on to tapping point 7, under the nose. Tap with two fingers and say out loud as you tap:

"This remaining pain in my body is hard to let go of. I understand that it is a natural occurrence within my body. And my body does so much for me and functions so well that I will not blame my body for this pain. I will not blame my body for the way my energy flows."

Move on to tapping point 8, the chin. Tap with two fingers and say out loud as you tap:

"I love and accept that my body responds this way. I profoundly love and accept myself, even with this pain that I am feeling. I profoundly love and accept every single part of myself even with all of this pain. And although I am now ready to let go of the pain, I know that even if I don't let it go that I still completely love and accept every part of myself."

Move on to tapping point 9, the collarbone. You can tap on either side with all four fingers. Switch sides when you go through the tapping sequence the second time. Say out loud as you tap:

"But I am ready to let go of this remaining pain. I do not need it anymore. I can feel the pain leaving my body and I can feel the calm and peace coming into my body. I know this feeling of peacefulness. I know this feeling of calm. And I embrace these feelings within me now."

Move on to tapping point 10, under your arm. Tap on either side with all four fingers. Switch sides when you go through the tapping sequence the second time. Say out loud as you tap:

"I may still feel pain within my body sometimes. I recognize it and I may feel it. But I will not criticize myself or my body for having this pain. I am choosing to just recognize that it is there and recognize how it feels. And it is OK. I love and accept myself even with this pain. I love and accept my body and all of the amazing things it does for me. And I love and accept myself enough to let the pain go."

Once you've been through this tapping sequence twice, rate your pain again on a scale of 1 to 10. Do you notice some relief? My own experience has been that using this sequence in conjunction with the chakra clearing exercise contained in this book in the chapter about clearing the chakras can increase the relief experienced.

The most important thing to remember

EFT tapping has already helped thousands of people to resolve their emotional problems, get their energy flowing properly, and make huge and meaningful changes in their lives. I've personally seen people who I have done tapping sessions with turn every aspect of their lives around. I know one man who lost over 80 pounds in the months following his introduction to EFT tapping. I know a young woman who applied and was accepted to a prestigious college and became the first person ever in her family to get a degree. I've seen these incredible changes that people have made in their lives and *I want you to experience these amazing changes for yourself!*

I want you to be able to live the exact life you want, and achieve everything you want in life. But there is one last step I must share with you and it is the *single most important step* in this entire book. You have to actually *do* what you have learned. Just reading this book and then putting it down and forgetting about it is not enough. If this is what you do, your life will not change and you will be taking a pass on all the amazing opportunities that are waiting for you.

EFT tapping is not just something you learn. It is something you *do*. If you are serious about putting EFT tapping to work in your life, you must make tapping sequences a regular part of your life. When you feel the stress or anxiety becoming overwhelming, when you have a problem you feel you can't solve, when you have an argument with a friend, or when you face some challenge that seems insurmountable. In all these situations, it is not enough to just remember the things contained in this book. You must actually *make the time to apply the techniques*. To sit down, take ownership over your health and well-being, and apply the tapping sequence you now know.

I believe in you and I know you can succeed, even in the face of the darkest adversity.

One final note...

I love helping people. It is my greatest passion in life and I love to know when something I shared with someone was able to help them in their own life, even if only a little bit. If you enjoyed reading this book I would be extremely grateful if you could take just a minute or two of your time and write a review online on Amazon or on social media. I personally read all reviews and they help me to make my future books even better. Thank you so much for your support and again, all my very best wishes in getting everything you want out of life and more!

Yours,
Randal P. Lawrence

My free gift to you:

Thank you and congratulations on your purchase! To say thank you, I would like to give you a free instructional video that demonstrates how to tap. You can use this video as an aid while you progress through this book. To claim your free gift now please visit my website at the URL below. I hope you find the video helpful:

www.randallawrence.com

More books from Randal Lawrence

Available on Amazon:

EFT Tapping and the Law of Attraction
How to eliminate negativity and attract wealth, happiness, love, positivity, and abundance into your life starting TODAY!

EFT Tapping for Weight Loss
Overcome junk food cravings, increase your willpower, speed up your metabolism, and transform your mind and body!

EFT Tapping Miracles for the Soul:
Six inspiring and uplifting stories of positive change and transformation through Emotional Freedom Therapy tapping

Learn EFT Tapping NOW! Complete Beginner's Manual:
Relieve stress and anxiety, lose weight, control cravings and addictions, boost your confidence and self-esteem and attract abundance starting today

Printed in Great Britain
by Amazon.co.uk, Ltd.,
Marston Gate.